I0095322

Rescuing Jill

How MDMA, with a Dash of Mushrooms, Healed My Childhood Trauma-Induced PTSD

Jill Sitnick

This work recounts events in the author's life as truthfully as childhood memories allow. Occasionally, dialogue was edited for readability. All names and locations have been changed or omitted except for my pets. They need all the fame they can get.

ISBN: 979-8-9860226-0-4

Cover design by: Klassic Designs
Library of Congress Control Number: 2022906408
Printed in the United States of America

CONTENTS

Introduction

Do Epic Shit

MDMA and magic mushrooms saved my life. Can they save yours? I don't know. But I have a hunch that if you picked up this book, there is something, somewhere, in the back of your brain, or your body, telling you there is a problem.

Or maybe you know someone who is deeply sad and lonely.

I have a little sign on my desk that reads *Do Epic Shit*. That sign is there to remind me to do things my way, especially when my way is a bit different from what other people would do. In my career and my life, I've made some decisions that became *Epic Shit* fast.

- Having a relationship with a man who gave me over twenty years of love, laughter, and constant support. *Epic Shit.*
- Getting recruited into Big Tech from a small K12 district and winning the highest sales award for outstanding work. *Epic Shit.*
- No longer qualifying for a childhood trauma-induced PTSD diagnosis and sharing my often-embarrassing trauma healing journey to help others. *Epic Shit.*

I wrote this book for you. I wrote this book to show there is a path to healing deep childhood trauma.

- If you feel emotions in your body that show themselves as physical pain and discomfort, then you might have some trauma making itself known to you.
- Are you hyper-vigilant and constantly looking over your shoulder because you know something terrible is coming?
- Do you know it is just a matter of time until life throws you another devastating blow from which you'll need to recover?
- Do you have a deep sense of isolation because you know you aren't worth loving?

Those are just a few hints that you have some trapped emotions from childhood trauma. There are more symptoms, but these are the ones I experienced the most.

So here is what I have done for you in the following pages: I've described for you my one-year healing story that spanned three psychedelic-assisted psychotherapy sessions. I told the story as it happened so you could discover, just as I did, how the therapy worked. I avoided as much 20/20 hindsight as possible to give you a realistic description of the work involved and the blind spots that trauma gave me as I experienced them.

My healing wasn't a straight road, and you'll see the twists and turns as I did the arduous work.

My early readers often gave me feedback along the lines of, "Your parents' behavior wasn't your fault."

That was exactly what my trauma didn't let me see or believe.

If at times, you are talking back to this book with what you know to be obvious, then you have hit on exactly how trauma impacts young brains. As trauma-carrying adults, we can see the correct roles of parents and children in other people's lives.

But darned if we see, or more importantly, *feel* those correct roles in our own lives.

In staying true to my story as it unfolded, I think I should give you the three biggest *hindsight is 20/20* hints to make your reading more enjoyable.

First Hint: This healing took work! Firefighters who run toward the flames are heroes. Anyone who goes toward his or her internal pain is also a hero. This shit was hard. Fucking hard. I had a year of feeling terrible, lonely, sad, heartbroken, and angry. Sometimes my emotions were just under the surface while I was at work, and other times they exploded while I did tasks around the house. I made the most progress when I was present with the shitty feelings and memories that surfaced from my subconscious.

I did not know the level of dedication this healing required. The psychedelics and my doctors, who prefer to be called **guides** in my story, were the supporting players while I ran the bases. I had to do the work. I had to be willing to run towards the pain. I had to remember horrible memories, that the MDMA let me see without my body reacting in fear, that I had locked away long ago.

My therapist gave me the approximate breakdown of the work around this therapy. I think it shows how 80% of the work relies on the patient doing the hard work:

40% = Talk therapy
20% = Medicated with psychedelics
40% = Integrating new perspectives into life

Second Hint: This book is not a trip report. Instead, I show you my specific healing moments. In my first two journeys with MDMA, which is described as a *relational psychedelic*, my healing happened in the months of integration *after* the medicated journeys. There weren't any stereotypical visuals when I was medicated with MDMA. There was a lot, and I mean *a lot,* of conversation with my internal voice and my guides. I'm a chatty person so that's how the medicine worked for me.

Integrating these journeys into my life meant that childhood memories had to be remembered and analyzed from an adult perspective instead of the usual way I had viewed them – as a traumatized child. Consequently, I wrote about some horrible memories so you could see the shift in how I thought about them. Shifting my perspectives and opinions about those traumatic memories was the key to my success.

With that said, if you think reading about the abuse I experienced could cause you to be uncomfortable, then you can skip most of those memories. You'll see I formatted them with ●●●●●●● before and after. Some of my perspective shifts might not be as clear, but you can absolutely skip my accounts of abuse and horrible life events and understand how this therapy worked for me.

Third Hint: My third journey, which incorporated MDMA and psilocybin (magic mushrooms), happened because I had hit a wall in my healing. I had a major trauma point that needed massive restructuring in my mind. I'm not a doctor and can't speak to the neuroscience at play here. All I know is magic mushrooms stepped in and with some amazing visuals, they let me craft new thinking about my childhood. I allow you in the sidecar of the healing process by sharing some of the transcripts from that third journey so you can see the healing as it happened while I was medicated.

That third journey's healing put into perspective all the pain and child-centric view of my life during the prior year's work. I know I felt relieved that all my fear-filled emotions finally made sense!

I have lots of hopes for readers who take the time to walk a year of my life with me.

- I hope my story shines a light on a therapy that can help other people living with PTSD.
- I hope I have combatted the ridiculous stigma around psychedelics that generations were incorrectly fed.
- I hope lawmakers realize the amazing opportunity in front of us and allow compounds to be reclassified for continued research into psychedelic-assisted psychotherapy.

I know my life would have been much less painful if this therapy had been available when I was in my twenties. My mother told me that she had wasted her life on her death bed. If this treatment had been available, she might have had a fighting chance at a happy life. Heck, she might have been able to become the lawyer she always dreamed of being.

It is my deepest hope that this book gives a voice to the next generation of people living with PTSD who need the option of this kind of therapy.

Chapter 1

Fucking Clichés

My healing journey using psychedelic psychotherapy for childhood trauma-induced PTSD started with the death of my partner, Carl. After twenty years of sharing a laughter-filled, loving life with him, I was bereft.

I had lost my most favorite person.

Carl's enthusiasm for life and adventure had been infectious. Our life together was a wonderful blend of perfectly timed sarcastic comments and holding hands while watching movies. We were equally happy getting purposely lost during our travels or hanging out reading on the couch. We had our own language, and as with many long-term relationships, we often finished each other's sentences. I felt safe and loved with him. With Carl I always belonged, and I knew he would always be there for me.

Until he wasn't.

His battle with bladder cancer ended unexpectedly when he passed away at home in his sleep one night.

While I was thankful that his death was quick, and that he wasn't hooked up to a myriad of beeping machines, his sudden death crushed my heart and spirit. I had prepared for taking care of him as he fought the disease. I hadn't prepared for the silence in the house after the black funeral parlor hearse drove away.

The days after his death were a blur of tears and intense feelings that half of me was gone. With the help of my amazing friends, who rotated visits to keep me fed and made sure I didn't sink into a deep depression, I was functioning again in about two weeks.

But I wasn't living normally.

When I went back to work, it took all my energy to focus on every task. I worked in big tech with a job that required travel, and I remember long car rides where I took advantage of the many miles and cried from rest stop to rest stop. While in the initial stages of my grief, I realized that my anxiety, anger, and fear of the future oozed through my *polite society* filters. I said what I thought about life's unfairness way too often. This wasn't a behavior someone in a customer service role for universities should engage in.

On one of those early work trips to Penn State, I remember canceling a work dinner with coworkers because I couldn't get my tears under control. Every time I cleaned myself up and tried to look presentable, a wave of anger and tears would take me back to huddling in my hotel room with the box of tissues.

My anger got worse as the weeks went by. My life's partner-in-crime was gone, and I couldn't stem the flood of rage I felt at the universe. I got quite a few raised eyebrows back then because my anger translated into biting comments about everything. I had zero tolerance for any shit.

One of my dear friends took me to dinner because that's what people did back then—they fed me. At a lovely Italian restaurant, I angrily ranted, through tears, about something so monumentally stupid that I don't remember it. I felt like all my nerve endings were exposed and on fire back then. Everything was a red alert, level 10! My cursing got us a few curious looks from folks at nearby tables.

He calmly texted me his therapist's number. Mentally, I gave that contact a middle finger. When my friend saw my hesitation, he looked me in the eye and said it was ok to get help. He asked me to try it since he had done great work with this doctor. I didn't think I had anything left to lose in my grief, so I agreed to call.

It was the right decision.

I drove to her Philadelphia office and liked that I got to visit a part of the city I didn't see too often. Within about five minutes of introducing myself, I was a bundle of tears. She was a petite woman sitting across from me in what looked like a super comfortable chair, and she let me cry. The couch I was sitting on was safe. Her office was safe. Her presence was safe. I could show my fear and sadness without her trying to make it ok with some platitude. She let my emotions unfold in front of her.

I finally pulled myself together enough to chat a bit. I shared how Carl had been so important to me, and I didn't know how to function without him. In her wisdom, she gave me a zombie analogy to explain how partners grieve. She said I was learning to walk after losing a leg while dealing with the gaping stab wound of his death. Her point was clear; I had to give myself time to grieve, heal, and learn how to live differently. Her advice and demeanor during that first meeting kept me coming back. She had allowed me to share all the feelings that made my friends uncomfortable. Plus, she matched my wit and wasn't afraid to be blunt when I needed it.

The main reason I thought I was there was to deal with grief—profound, blinding grief that robbed me of time and all caring. But the very first time we met, once I got myself under control, I also focused on getting my *polite society* filter back in place to avoid offending anyone. I felt disconnected from everything, and my widow's fog dampened my ability to think critically. It's called widow's fog for a reason, and it coated my entire life. I barely planned beyond a few hours, and weirdly, it took extra energy even to move. The fog had a mental and physical heaviness, and I struggled to focus and organize my thoughts for several months. Since I couldn't think straight, I blurted out too many thoughts that used to stay locked in my head. I thought I was letting my *meanness* show. I thought I was serving hater-aid juice to everyone.

Showing people the real me was dangerous. People couldn't know what was in my head. I had lived my life working to make sure people never got angry at me. I couldn't have explained it, but I was always convinced that if I angered someone, that person would make me a target. This was something I *knew* so deeply that I never pushed back against this belief. And I never questioned it. It just made sense that people would actively try to harm me if I upset them somehow.

Plus, I had always known I was a mean person at my core. I didn't know why. I couldn't pinpoint the moment I knew I was mean. I was only aware of my defect—my meanness. I usually hid my meanness by not saying what would pop into my head. I could be judgmental to the point of cutting and had learned that my quick wit could rub people the wrong way. I always appreciated when I met verbally quick people who liked to joke around because I could relax a bit and feel more comfortable. But most of the time, I worked hard to suppress the side of me that I defined as mean.

I was sure the only reason I had friends was that they didn't know the real me. I didn't understand why I felt that way; it was just something I knew. I didn't want anyone to know that I was an awful person who had kept myself well hidden under layers of politeness my whole life.

Fucking Clichés

I was a waterfall of sad tears washing away my new therapist's tissue supply. I had to learn how to process the worst grief I had ever felt while getting my survival tactics back in place to function professionally and stay financially safe. Sitting on her couch was one of the ways I worked to get my shit together so I didn't wind up with a pink slip from work.

Getting a great therapist was the first step on this unexpected winding journey. I didn't know that my grief would point me in a direction that would heal childhood trauma. All I knew was that my most favorite person was no longer by my side.

Carl's death was the fucking door that closed a part of my life I cherished. Meeting my new therapist to work through my grief was the new door that opened to help me with the next phase of my life.

Chapter 2

Panic Attacks Suck

For eighteen months I managed to survive my most profound grief with the best advice I got from one of my best friends who also had lost a partner.

There are no shoulds.

There—it was that simple. There was no rule book I had to follow to survive my heavy grief. I look back now at how lonely and desperate I was to find glimmers of escape from the chronic crushing pain.

Unfortunately, the haze of my widow's fog made work tasks take three times as long, so I racked up lots of hours, and quite a few vanilla-scented candles in the dark hours, as I tried to keep my head above water in my home office. I worked for a big technology company, and work was my lifeline.

It appeared I was adulting well. I continued to win sales awards at work, and my customers didn't know they were dealing with someone working through deep grief. I continued to make sound financial decisions to protect myself from uncertainty. The pets were healthy and filled the house with barks and squawks. My dog, Sadie, is a brown and white terrier mix with an adorable, white-tipped tail and floppy ears that bounce when she walks. She is known far and wide as Stinky Butt, Pooper Head, and Wackadoodle. My adopted, completely spoiled Indian Ringneck Parakeet, Kasha, was a blue and orange little asshole who ruled the house with ear-splitting screams and an "I deserve ALL the food, ALL the time" attitude.

I was a nightly boot camper who hoped that jumping jacks and push-ups could keep me occupied and not think of my house without Carl in the evenings. Everything on the surface looked great!

Inside, I was empty.

I especially struggled as I entered my second year of grief. Carl wasn't going to be in any future, and every second-year event cruelly reminded me of his absence. I was still a walking zombie, and I coped by keeping my crazy work hours and booking lots of work travel. The pace finally caught up with me via a vicious combination of strep and mono.

On one trip from Philadelphia to Pittsburgh and then State College, I came down with a strep infection. I just thought I caught a bad cold because I had grown up a relatively healthy kid and didn't understand the signs my body was sending. I figured a bad sore throat and my loss of appetite would go away in a few days.

When I left Pittsburgh and got to State College, I was three days in without any solid food and in such bad shape that I went to a 24-hour clinic. Unfortunately, their strep test came back negative, and I remember crying in frustration. There was nothing they could do for me. I finally got them to realize the pain my throat was causing me, and I hadn't slept and eaten anything solid for days. Thankfully, they gave me a pain killer and an antibiotic prescription.

I canceled my meetings and drove home as soon as the sun rose the following day. I drove the entire ride with a window open to ensure the chilly winter air kept me awake since I wasn't sure how the protein shakes I had bought at the local drug store and painkillers would mix.

As soon as I got close to home, I filled the prescription.

Without even returning the rental car, I headed home, took my medicine, and went right to bed.

In the middle of the night, I woke up to full body hives from my body's reaction to the onslaught of medication. I struggled to decide my next step as I looked at myself in the mirror. I thought long and hard about simply going back to bed and letting the reaction close my throat. I could just sink away from the pain that had been chronically following me for five days at this point. I wasn't thinking beyond the next decision – that's how exhausted I was mentally and physically. While looking at myself, my world's perspective focused on one decision; live or passively die by crawling back in bed.

This was the first time that my pets kept me alive. While Sadie was still at the kennel, my little asshole, Kasha, was downstairs covered and snug in her cage. I couldn't even think of her being rehomed again. Who would put up with her shit?

I got my ass to the emergency room.

I didn't answer the "Have you felt suicidal?" question very well during my intake process. The nurse gave me the side-eye when I said, "Well, I decided to drive here instead of die at home, so I guess that means something." I remember an awkward silence as I sat back, closed my eyes, and dreaded swallowing. I hadn't eaten anything solid for days, had only slept a few hours, my throat was a cylinder of knives, and I didn't have anyone at home anymore.

After assessing my condition, the ER doctor said to me, "You have a serious infection. We can fix you up if you want to be fixed up." He looked me straight in the eye and waited for an answer.

His bluntness cut through my hazy mind. Was it worth it

to get fixed up only to keep "zombie-ing" my way through life, or was I going to wake up and start living again? Would my beneficiaries have great vacations or buy fast cars because I didn't take care of myself, or was I going to live?

With what fleeting energy I still had, I gave the doctor my best *I'm ready to live again* nod.

That hospital stay was like a huge fan that blew away some of the widow's fog. After four bed-bound days where Jell-O became my stomach's best friend, I was released and had to fight the worst exhaustion I had ever felt. It turned out that not only did I have strep, but I had also contracted mono.

I strictly followed my prescription and supplement regime for weeks to regain my energy that mono had stolen. I finally got my trophy for choking down horse pills by being able to stay awake all day after about six weeks. My widow's fog dissipated even more, and I decided to think seriously about a relationship instead of the drive-by dating I had done to distract myself from my grief. After a few mishaps, I met a lovely man who became one of my best friends and my second longest romantic relationship.

Everything seemed to be on track. I had battled my way back to semi-normalcy.

But then, everything went to shit.

The most ordinary of ordinary things happened. I got a work email about new certification requirements for folks like me in sales. I had been recruited from my twenty years in a K12 to a big technology company, in the education sector, and cloud computing was the cool kid on the block. Since I wasn't in a technical support role, I never expected to need certifications to keep my job. And frankly, I wasn't interested in technology infrastructure. When customers would ask me a deep technical question, I would find them a better resource. I'd always been focused on technology use for increased learning outcomes. I had zero interest in the back-end infrastructure that made the magic in the classroom happen. In my career back in my school district's tech department, I had my fill of plugging in CAT5 cables to make servers come to life.

When I finished reading that email, that to me signaled my job responsibilities were going to change in a direction I didn't want; a police siren screamed in my head, my heart rate skyrocketed, and my palms were sweaty. I spiraled from having a great house and job to being unemployed and homeless in .03 seconds. I saw a rather ordinary email as the death knell to my career and life as I knew it. Just like a three-year-old not getting a candy bar at the checkout line, I went into a complete meltdown. I felt my heart pounding in my chest because *I knew* that tiny email was the end of my career. I don't know how I knew—I just knew! Not only that, but *I knew* I wasn't going to be employable ever again, and I would immediately plummet into poverty. I have no idea how *I knew* my life was essentially over. My body and mind felt like I was being chased by some wild animal that I couldn't outrun.

My friends, coworkers, and boyfriend told me everything would be fine. It wasn't like I couldn't kick the ass out of tests—that was my academic history. We won't talk about high school chemistry—I mean, there is a chart, for goodness sakes—why did I need to memorize it? My job wasn't fundamentally changing. The company just wanted sales folks to have a 100-level understanding of their technology. The requirement totally made sense.

But I couldn't get the fear out of my head.

I constantly reviewed my Plan Bs so that I wouldn't spiral

into homelessness. Both of my divorced parents, at various times, had thrown me out of their homes before I was eighteen. I knew how it felt to have rugs unexpectedly pulled out from under me. Consequently, I had built several financial safety nets to catch me in case of any emergency. I drove up my screen time when I checked my financial apps an embarrassing number of times each day.

I wasn't going to be homeless. I wasn't going to be living in my car with my pets. I wasn't going to be without food. It didn't matter if I did lose my job, which I wouldn't—I would be okay.

But my mind and body didn't listen to reason. That police siren in my head squealed for months while I was in hyper-alert flight/fight mode. My stomach was in knots, my left shoulder near my neck was on fire, and I didn't sleep well.

There was absolutely no logical reason for this constant, exhausting state of alert.

Out of frustration, I finally called my therapist. She always kindly let me pick up and put down therapy as my grief ebbed and flowed. To her credit, she jumped right in to dance with my panic. I attacked her tissue box again while I explained my months-long panic attack. My mind was like an Uber driver asking, "Are you sure?" about a destination that wasn't sketchy at all. I couldn't convince myself everything was fine. I could explain all the ways I would be safe, in a warm home, with the pets cuddled and well-fed as usual. But darned if I could calm myself down. My body constantly told me I was in danger.

I sat on my therapist's comfortable sofa, exhausted and bewildered because I couldn't calm the fuck down. It never occurred to me one bit that my behavior was linked to my childhood.

Chapter 3

No Trauma Here

As my therapist and I explored my never-ending panic attack, she asked me to describe my physical symptoms. I described my burning neck pain, bunched-up shoulders, and upset stomach. In the most stereotypical therapist way, she asked me to focus on my physical symptoms. She wanted to know what I thought my body was trying to tell me. I never thought about my "anxiety behaviors" as messengers. They were just part of my life.

I explained that my body was telling me I was in danger. I was always in peril; my body just told me to what degree by how badly my neck seared or my jaws clenched.

Then she went a step further when she asked me to try and remember times in my life when I felt those physical symptoms. I wasn't great at those answers because I often remembered my father's anger and abuse in a whitewashed *it happened over thirty years ago* kind of way. And really, I thought she was off the mark. I thought my body's reaction was a nasty case of imposter syndrome. I assumed my stress was because my boss would figure out any day now that he had hired someone who didn't know her shit!

Other than Carl, and one of my best friends, Kathy, I had never invited anyone to my childhood circus and introduced the clowns. I rarely discussed my childhood, and if I was pressed, I often quickly summarized it with three words: abuse, suicides, and drugs. Those words usually stopped people from asking further questions, so they worked well.

In one of our therapy sessions, I described an incident with my father when I was nine.

●●●●●●●

I remembered my father as a big man. He was about 6'2" and 230 pounds. I remember feeling overwhelmed by his size and the weight of his anger when he would beat me. One day my father was upset about something and was yelling at me in the kitchen. He suddenly left the room, but I was frozen in place because that was weird behavior. I rarely escaped getting hit when he was riled up, and I was afraid to move. This time, when he came back to the kitchen, he had a small travel bag with him. He pulled out pictures of my mother who had tried to commit suicide by slicing her wrists in the bathroom tub.

The image I remember most is of my mother's left arm on the side of the tub with its lines of blood that pooled on the tile floor.

●●●●●●●

With pride, I explained to my therapist how I calmly looked at those pictures and didn't respond to him. I can't even remember if I felt anything looking at those pictures. I didn't know why my father was showing them to me, but it seemed like some trap to get me to respond so he would have an excuse to keep yelling or hit me. So, I didn't respond. I got exceptionally good at not responding in general.

RESCUING JILL

My therapist's raised eyebrows stopped me mid-story. I hadn't seen someone's response to my father's cruelty in years, and I paused—embarrassed.

I had focused on my strategic reaction to avoid getting hit, while she focused on my father's overt cruelty. First, it meant he took Kodak film pictures of my mother after she had sliced her wrists and had passed out in a tub of her blood, got them developed at a photography store (this was the 1970s), and showed his nine-year-old daughter those pictures years later. But it was just one of the many weird and cruel things my father did, which to me was just a big pile of ugliness. I felt a familiar flush of shame on my cheeks as I realized, *uh, here is more shit about my childhood; now she knows I'm fucked up. Normal people don't grow up like this. I'll never be like normal people.*

As we explored the roots of my physical symptoms and anxiety, more and more memories, that I hadn't thought about in years, spewed out. I didn't enjoy going down memory lane, and my tight shoulders and upset stomach were physical reminders of how I felt as a child. Those were the symptoms I felt before and after the beatings. I have a distinct memory of huddling in the corner of my room, maybe when I was nine, and I was so angry I couldn't make the beatings stop. My neck was on fire because I couldn't think my way out of my life. That neck pain became my signal that I was trapped and in danger.

And when I talked about my father, my face tensed up like I had just caught a whiff of a baby's dirty diaper. I finally felt comfortable showing how much my father disgusted me in the safety of my therapist's office.

My therapist tiptoed into my PTSD diagnosis. She had me explain where I experienced the unpleasant emotions in my body. I would point to my shoulder when I described

19

work drama. I could feel my stomach contract when I remembered childhood beatings. My posture would go rigid when I explained any threat to my security. Yet, I resisted when my therapist explained that I was responding to childhood trauma. I certainly didn't believe I had PTSD.

I reasoned that I had just overreacted to life's stressors or was going through another stage in my grief work. I felt ashamed that I took things so seriously all the time. There must have been something wrong with my brain for my thoughts to keep spiraling. My childhood wasn't any worse and a darned bit better than others—so no—I couldn't possibly have trauma. I was a functioning adult for goodness sakes—didn't she know that? Trust me; I tried to convince her as best I could that I didn't have PTSD.

But the reality was that I had been in her office for over two months by that point and was still terrified that my life, as I knew it, would be over. My one and only goal, since I was old enough to work, was to get financially secure enough so that no one could physically hurt me or leave me homeless. I only wanted security.

I had security out the wazzoo. I had paid off my house, had investments, and lived well below my means. No one could rip out all the various rugs I had in place!

In response to all of that planning and security, my body was still in a non-stop panic attack because it felt I would be homeless in a month. I knew in my logical brain that it couldn't happen in a month, but I couldn't tell my body to relax and stop feeling like I was running for my life.

I kept repeating in my therapy sessions how much danger I felt in between describing childhood memories and reviews of my overall security. I would list all my Plan Bs and then return to my dread because I *knew* something evil was right around the corner that I couldn't predict. I was an anxious wreck about what was sure to be the next bomb the universe would throw at me.

My therapist gently pointed out that I seemed stuck. She said that she had seen my healing progress with my grief work. She didn't see that kind of progress here. She mentioned how often I talked about the same thing—having life suddenly shift below my feet and leave me starting over from scratch while living in my car with a clingy dog and a cheeky parrot.

I was like, "Of course, I keep repeating myself—you do not understand how much the universe is after me!"

Finally, my therapist assigned me some reading. While I probably had enough trauma to pay off her mortgage, she wanted me to move a little faster. She tried to tell me my body's "check engine" light had been on for years while I ignored it and that it was a trauma response to be *stuck* in a way of thinking.

She suggested I read, *The Body Keeps the Score* by Dr. Bessel van der Kolk, and I picked it up after reading the reviews. The book didn't disappoint. I realized my brain had responded to traumatic events by the last page, and the unhealed emotions were "pinned" in my brain. Dr. van der Kolk explained, "Trauma is trapped emotions from a bad time."

That book showed that I responded normally to the abuse I suffered as a child. My body and brain had become unable to distinguish between normal *I can't find my keys* stress and life-threatening danger. I reacted to both equally. This was an uncontrollable, instinctive response that my mind had developed as a survival strategy, which kept me safe as a child. It had served an important function and was evidence of my mind and body caring about and protecting me. Only now, the same strategies that helped protect me in childhood were no longer serving a useful purpose.

I saw myself in that book. I saw my parents. I saw my physical trauma responses. Why couldn't I stop my deep, burning neck pain with meditation when I felt threatened? Why did my throat tighten and my chest get heavy when I started to hope for something? Why was I constantly overthinking in a hyper-vigilant fearful mental state with my jaw clenched?

Dr. van der Kolk wrote, "Trauma comes back as a reaction, not a memory." His book helped me understand that my body reacted to everyday stress, like when I suffered abuse. Most importantly, that book showed that I responded *normally* to the abuse.

I finally understood my physical responses to stress were not abnormal—they were trauma responses. I also understood that other successful adults had their parents' abusive voices in their heads. My trauma responses couldn't heal in a mindfulness program getting my ass sore from sitting silently for eight hours. Nor could my sky-high heart rate during boot camp clear my head enough to take away my constant fear.

I finally saw the PTSD symptoms as symptoms. I finally saw the possibility of help getting to deal with my parents' shit.

I had taken the first step to heal; I admitted I had childhood trauma-induced PTSD.

Chapter 4

I'm Done Fighting

After I blasted through Dr. Bessel van der Kolk's book, my therapist and I talked about psychedelic-assisted psychotherapy. This was about two months from when I had first reached out about my panic attack. She explained that our nervous systems can create a myriad of mental and physical health symptoms in response to trauma and that psychedelics have been shown to disrupt those responses and let people release their trauma. I didn't have much experience with drugs, and my mind immediately pictured too much neon tie-dye for anyone's own good. I couldn't make the link between the stereotypes I had been media-fed my whole life to a therapy for PTSD. She smiled and assured me that I would see a different side to psychedelics with some research.

I had a healthy skepticism about mental health drugs and mental health professionals. I left her office without agreeing to the treatment for a few reasons.

First, my mother was clinically depressed her entire adulthood. Her prescriptions changed over the years, but they never balanced her "chemical imbalance." My mother's terrible experience with therapists made me almost ignore my friend's advice to get help right after Carl died.

Secondly, I was keenly aware of how chemicals could impact my thoughts. For instance, after my hospital visit, my mood sank to dangerous self-harm levels when I took steroids. Nothing but concern for my pets stopped me from slicing my wrists in the tub. I had a lifetime tutorial from the scars on my mother's arms on how to kill myself.

My neighbor, a nurse, saw me ugly crying when I walked my dog, Sadie. I told her about my prescriptions, and she pointed her finger at me and said, "All your emotions are from the steroids. No life decisions! This will be over by Tuesday. Promise me!"

I did promise. I waited until Tuesday. I am forever thankful.

Lastly, I had discounted psychedelic therapy when I had heard rumblings about it on Tim Ferris's podcast, *The Tim Ferris Show*. At the time, I felt an ayahuasca experience, which would entail drinking a psychedelic brew in a foreign country, could be dangerous. I wasn't going to trust my brain to chemicals and people I didn't know. My brain had got me through life. I wasn't going to make it vulnerable to chemicals I didn't understand. My research had stopped before it even started.

But like the good student that I am, I did my research homework the next day after my session. I went to MAPS.org, the Multidisciplinary Association for Psychedelic Studies site. I read about their PTSD and MDMA research. According to the site, patients only needed a few treatments for their symptoms to subside. That was the best news I had ever read about mental injuries. (I had started to think about my brain's responses to my childhood trauma as mental injuries —not illness.) Suddenly, I saw a viable option to heal. I felt that my brain had been bruised by traumatic events that needed the right medicine. Just my personal distinction was a step in the right direction in my healing. It was the starting point for me to face the shame I carried that I was defective for not getting over my parents' shit.

A quick Google search also led me to work at Johns Hopkins, which legitimized psychedelic treatment for mental health even more.

After looking at those sites, I was about 90% convinced.

Here's what I don't like to admit—and will probably surprise my friends—I was at the end of my rope. I had achieved my only goal of being financially self-sufficient. I wasn't "retire in the islands" wealthy or anything, but I wouldn't wind up homeless. I had things well set up, yet I combed financial tips every day because I thought I must have missed something. I had this nagging, ever-present thought that I wasn't safe. My trauma had rewired my brain to protect me, so I was always on alert. I didn't know how to relax and live differently.

My certification-inspired panic attack had raged for months into an overthinking hell from which I couldn't escape. Yet part of my mind knew that my overthinking was ridiculous. The last twenty years of my life have been stable. Once I got away from my parents and got my first teaching job, my world settled into a safe work routine, cooking (well, really baking), house cleaning, and Friday date nights with a lovely man. Yet the raging panic attack and physical symptoms couldn't *see* those years or the proof that life would be good. If my own life wasn't good enough to calm me down, what would?

My conservative financial portfolio also couldn't take away the fear. I was bone-tired of constantly looking over my shoulder for the next threat that would wipe me out financially. A few times in my therapy sessions, I said, "I'm done. If the universe craps all over me again and leaves me with nothing, like it has done so many times before, I'm out. I'm done fighting against it."

I was an incredibly successful, financially independent

pet parent who was borderline suicidal. I was tired of running a fear-powered race that didn't seem to have a finish line. My body and internal fear didn't *see* the last twenty years of happiness and success. My trauma didn't *see* the beautiful life I had with Carl to know that the future was safe.

I was living trapped in the trauma of my childhood.

I couldn't envision a future for myself.

I understood that I needed to do something different to find happiness moving forward. My adult brain was saying, *Yo, calm the fuck down. Everything is fine. You are safe.* Meanwhile, my body was "talking" through my physical symptoms (anxiety attacks) from my childhood trauma, saying, *Yo, time to armor up; shit is about to go down.*

The exhaustion I felt was the last 10% of the decision. I was so tired of constantly armoring up for battle. I was dangerously close to giving up the fight.

Chapter 5

40%-20%-40%

In our next session, I told my therapist I was ready to try psychedelic-assisted psychotherapy. She explained the therapeutic protocol and how she and a guide (who was also a doctor) would work with me.

1. She screened me to ensure there was no history of schizophrenia in my family. Since I had been going to her for years at this point, she knew my only diagnosis was PTSD. I certainly had anxiety, but my self-soothing behaviors (hair twirling, lip biting) were on display because of my PTSD.

2. I needed to stop using Wellbutrin well before the journey to be safe.

3. 40% of the entire process was our pre-journey talk therapy sessions. Understanding the feelings underneath my PTSD symptoms was the first hurdle. Creating my intentions, or mindset, for the journey was a prime focus during these therapy sessions. Those intentions were fundamental because she said, "Your outcomes will align with your intentions."

4. The next step, or 20% of the process, was my medicinal journey using MDMA. MDMA is a synthetic drug whose full name is 3,4-Methylenedioxymethamphetamine. It was synthesized in the early 1900s and had been used in

27

mental health research before being classified as a Schedule 1 drug in the drug wars of the 80s. MDMA doesn't produce the neon-shaped visuals that are often associated with psychedelics. I describe MDMA as a relationship drug because it increased my trust in my doctors, calmed my body down when I thought about scary memories, and allowed me to show myself some empathy.

5. The remaining 40% of the process would be my integration which starts after the journey and could last for days, weeks, and even months. I was a little fuzzy about that part, so my therapist explained it is a little like physical therapy. I would have to do work at home dealing with my memories and looking at them through the lens of my adult perspective. I would also be checking in with my therapist and guide according to my schedule. Most importantly, she encouraged me to start journaling, even when I might not feel like journaling, because she warned me that perspective shifts could be subtle, and I might miss them if I didn't take time for myself and journal.

I read that traveling metaphors of *trips* and *journeys* are linked with psychedelic use. My therapist used the word *journey* to describe our day together while I was to be medicated. She explained a guide's role in psychedelic-assisted psychotherapy could range from simply sitting and being a sober companion with a patient going *inward* to guiding a patient through difficult memories or experiences.

I was surprised that the MDMA, usually referred to as the "medicine," would be in my system for only one-fifth of my entire therapeutic process. I had heard on various podcasts the exuberant claims that therapeutic journeys were like ten years of therapy in five hours. Here my therapist told me there would be months of work on both sides of my medicinal journey to get results.

She assured me I would get all the support I needed. She didn't think I was defective or broken. She made it clear I was a whole person who could heal.

With that, we started seriously mapping how my body reacted to the emotions I still felt from painful childhood memories.

Chapter 6

Ugly Crying

This is the part of my story where one of my best friends, Kathy, had a crystal ball. While it was the start of this healing journey for me, she knew I was a wounded little girl wrapped up in adult layers.

Kathy and I met when I was in my early twenties when I worked at one of those shit jobs that fueled my need to get a college education. She gave me a ton of free help when she worked on her counseling degree. Because I was still terrified of my father, I was a counseling student's dream subject. She even administered eye movement desensitization and reprocessing (EMDR) treatment that stopped one of my recurring nightmares.

●●●●●●●●

The nightmare came from when I was a toddler, and my father charged up the stairs like a bull elephant and dragged me down the steps by my right leg. He threw me across the room, and I hit my head on the opposite wall. He charged up the stairs to beat my mother while I stayed downstairs and tried to make myself as small as possible. This crucial memory never got dusty – it has stayed with me my entire life.

After the EMDR therapy, I remembered his

predatory scowl as he came up the stairs, but the image no longer scared me. I saw it from my adult perspective as someone he could no longer abuse. It was like one of my childhood Scratch and Sniff stickers that had lost its smell. It was just another part of my childhood. I didn't get flushed or scared when I remembered it. Most importantly, I never dreamed of that horrible night ever again.

●●●●●●●●

While we sat on Kathy's deck with the night's cool ocean breeze, I told her about the planned MDMA journey. She was curious and had a bunch of questions I couldn't answer. But because it was Kathy—I shared my fear of messing up. As I cuddled deeper into a throw to combat the night air, I admitted I was scared. What if my intentions were wrong? What if I couldn't do whatever one does while on a journey? What if the therapy didn't work? What then? What if "Jill, who always does an excellent job, doesn't do an excellent job?" I remember ugly crying because I was scared I would fuck up and waste everyone's time.

And you know what she said? She said my fear was about me trying to stay safe.

Safe from what? Safe from whom?

She said my inner five-year-old was still scared of adults. That stopped me. I gave it some thought and then wholly discounted it—I only associated memories of my mother's suicide attempt when I was five. The EMDR and thirty-ish years made most of my childhood memories hazy. I knew my childhood was crappy, but I didn't remember the day-to-day fear and dread as I did when I was in my twenties. Kathy didn't remember specifics, but she remembered her horror years ago when I had described my childhood. Plus, she had gotten a few A's on assignments by analyzing my trauma background.

The memory I most associated with my inner five-year-old was my mother's most serious suicide attempt. After several unsuccessful attempts, she again failed when she tried to shoot herself. That event was so huge that it eclipsed the paternal abuse. No one really seemed to look at why my mother went to this level and why a little girl had bitten lips, had nightmares, and had bald spots from pulling out her hair. My mother was blamed for my behavior. So her shotgun suicide attempt has always been the life event that I linked to that age.

Kathy reminded me of other childhood stories I told her that I had long banished to the "Shitty Early Childhood Memories—Don't Open" manilla folder in my brain. She remembered how I fearfully told her about my father locking me, a screaming toddler, outside in a lightning storm and laughing at me through the sliding patio door. She remembered my father taking me to see *Jaws* (I had months of nightmares). She remembered my stories of feeding myself because someone had to. She remembered how I described my anxiety-driven hair pulling, lip biting, and rocking at night. And more importantly, she recalled how terrified I was of him in my twenties.

But I didn't believe her. I hadn't opened that "Shitty Early Childhood Memories - Don't Open" manilla folder for over thirty years. I think it has an auto-delete function based on time because now, in middle age, my conscious mind remembers very little from that time. To me, that early age didn't seem to hold any power over me. I was far more concerned with traumas I could remember at sixteen and nineteen.

Kathy kept trying to convince me that all my trepidation was trapped emotions from when I experienced pain or abuse as a little girl. She said my inner five-year-old needed healing, but she was afraid and didn't think any adults could help. By agreeing to this therapy, I was having her, my inner five-year-old Jill, go into unknown territory without a safe word.

Spoiler Alert: Kathy was right. Everything would eventually circle back to my trauma when I was five.

But not like I would have guessed.

Chapter 7

First Journey Preparation

For several weeks before my first journey, my body and mind were on high alert. I rode some emotional roller coasters and made mountains out of molehills. I was exhausted because I tossed and turned at night. My self-soothing strategies of twirling my hair and biting my lips were front and center. These behaviors had always been part of my life, but they were dialed all the way up. My subconscious was terrified of what this therapy would do to me.

A week before my MDMA journey, my guides and I had a virtual meeting to help prepare my intentions for the journey. I met my guide and learned about his medical background and experience with psychedelic-assisted psychotherapy. At the end of that session, I felt extremely comfortable with his credentials. I also understood that my guide, and my therapist, would both guide and support me during the therapeutic journey.

At the time, I didn't understand the importance of "set and setting" with psychedelic-assisted psychotherapy. I've come to understand that "set" is the patient's mindset. When my therapist talked to me about being open to healing, I remembered a conversation I had with a nurse when I was hospitalized.

I was fully dressed and ready to leave the hospital at 9 AM on the day I was discharged. Anyone who has been discharged from a hospital knows it isn't a quick process. A kind nurse apologized for the delay at around 11 AM.

She said, "We can tell the patients who want to get better, and we know you are ready to go. We'll get you out of here as soon as we can."

My mindset at the hospital was a similar mindset getting ready for my therapeutic journey. I wanted to get better. My therapist and guide had answered every single one of my embarrassing questions (Would this be like an ayahuasca experience? Should I expect to throw up?), and their answers let me know I would be physically safe. Being able to focus on my intentions to heal put me in the right mindset. If I had been scared about any part of the process, I knew I would have been able to reschedule the journey.

Setting, to me, refers to the kind of place where a journey happens. Psychedelic-assisted psychotherapy journey rooms are often designed to be cozy instead of hospital sparse. I didn't know what the journey room would look like, but when my guide gave me a list of items to bring with me (warm socks, an eye mask, comfortable clothing), I asked if the room would have the thermostat set to teeth-chattering temperatures like all of Carl's hospital rooms. My guide chuckled and assured me I would find the journey room warm and inviting.

My intentions weren't expectations. Instead, my intentions were what I wanted to heal within my mind. My two intentions focused heavily on fear and, in hindsight, seem almost similar. But for me, the future was an antagonist in my life's own story. For me, those intentions were very separate and equally frightening.

I intended to:
- Stop being afraid of the future.
- Stop being afraid that the universe would punish

35

me whenever things were going well.

As scared and nervous as I was, I was also freaking excited! In preparation for the mid-September Thursday, I carefully formatted my intentions, double-checked them, and actually printed them (who prints anymore?), so they would look nice and neat. They were even highlighted red on my perfectly formatted sheet. I didn't take a walk to Type A Crazy Town and use a different font, but I was so excited about the day that I was *thisssss* close to doing so.

I showed up that unseasonably warm fall morning ready to go!

Chapter 8

Let's Go

The journey room, or setting, was an oasis from the hustle and bustle of life. There were beautiful tapestries on the walls and several sitting areas. It smelled faintly of sage, and I remember smiling when I saw a pile of blankets folded by the side of a neatly made-up mattress. My dog and I could win medals for our expert cuddling under warm *blankies*, and I always appreciate relaxing, fluffy blanket opportunities.

This was not a blinding fluorescent-lit hospital room like the dozens Carl and I had been assigned while he fought bladder cancer. We could practically taste the disinfectants as the sounds of never-ending digital beeps were our background as we chatted. Even the waiting rooms, where I spent the equivalent of weeks over the years, were cold and plastic. Comfort never was a priority for anyone involved. I'll never get over the irony that our most medically sophisticated hospitals can be so stark and frightening.

This room was like a cup of hot chocolate after coming in from the cold. I felt immediately welcomed.

So there I was, trying to be as polite as possible while trying not to be nervous while being terribly nervous. My guides and I took off our shoes, and we sat in one of the little sitting areas. I contributed some pink Rose of Sharon blooms from my home's front walkway to the space. I remember being a bit sad at how they had wilted in the car when I looked at what others had brought. There were little stones, pictures, and even an action figure or two. People had brought items of meaning to the space, which served to create a *this has been done before, I'm safe* feeling to the experience. There was a comfort in knowing people before me had shared their deepest fears and shame. Oddly, it was genuinely lovely knowing I was part of a community of people working toward healing. I made a mental note to bring something more permanent than flowers if I found myself in this journey space ever again.

We then started the day with me sharing my parent's wedding album to give my guides some visual references. I don't have many pictures from my childhood, and I couldn't find any with or of my father. I didn't remember if we never had photos taken together or if I had trashed them over the years. Either way, the wedding album held the only images I could find of my parents together.

With a classic 1960s white hair bow that contrasted with her black shoulder-length hair, my mother rarely smiled in those pictures. Standing next to my father, who was 6'3" she seemed delicate with her 5'5" slim frame. Looking at those pictures reminded me that I inherited my slightly crooked smile from my mother and my thirty-three-inch inseam legs from my father.

My guides' perspectives about the album were fascinating. They didn't see any joy in those mid-1960s cardboard-backed pictures. I looked at those pictures again, and instead of just noticing how young they looked, it was the first time I saw my parents as scared adults on a big day. They were trying to do their best with what they had been emotionally given. Interestingly, my mother, and her parents, looked morose throughout most of the album. I had never caught that before since I always thought my mother looked sad. There is not one picture of my mother's parents smiling in that album. It was another slight hint that my mother had her own issues that weren't related to me at all.

Then we talked about my intentions to ensure there weren't more layers to my goals. We reviewed my fears of the future and the universe. As my guide and therapist passed the sage to bring good, healthy energy into the room, I stared at the two MDMA capsules. They looked like ordinary vitamins. I desperately wanted this treatment to do anything to make living life better. If those two tiny gray capsules could help, I was in!

My inner five-year-old wasn't.

Chapter 9

Chatty Jilly

After almost forty minutes after taking the MDMA capsules, I still sat comfortably in the sitting area. Once, a former coworker joked with me when she found me working on my laptop while seated on the board room floor. She said she was sure I could work for hours if I could "pop a squat" on the floor to work. She was right!

I was a happy camper just leaning against the wall hugging my legs. At some point I had closed my eyes, and I had a fantastic internal conversation. I heard an inner strong female voice telling me it was time for me to live! I kept describing her as a "strong, snarky woman." I had a classic best friend "pick me up" conversation in my head. I listened to someone who was entirely in my corner. She told me to start living for my happiness. (I didn't know it was my inner voice. I had never listened to my gut or inner voice before. I was that disconnected from my wants and needs.)

I didn't see this voice or have any neon-tinged visuals since MDMA is an empathogen that makes users feel empathetic and friendly towards others and themselves. There are blogs dedicated to arguing if MDMA should even be considered a psychedelic because it doesn't produce visuals during journeys. I'm not a doctor, and I'll never play one on TV, so I'll lean to the side of not caring about how it is classified. In my case, it connected me to my subconscious because I needed to be more empathetic toward myself. I felt fine physically, and my easily upset stomach stayed calm. At the time, I felt like the medicine in my system was communicating with me the way I most easily communicated—verbally.

I chatted fluently with my guides. My guides told me I wouldn't remember much of the actual journey, so they used one of their phones to record the session. Months later, when I heard the recordings, I learned I was noticeably clear when I communicated. I didn't slur my words as I do with too many margaritas. I also didn't lie. I simply didn't mention anything I didn't want to say, so any polite lies I had told throughout my life when people asked about my childhood—weren't told. The guides could ask me any question, and they were either going to get the truth or I would not share.

About ninety minutes into the session, my guides invited me to lie down and get comfortable. This procedure didn't dull my intellect or conversation skills. But doing anything other than occasionally getting up to use the restroom was off the table. I finally understood why the lovely mattress was so close to the sitting area. I didn't need help getting to the mattress, but if it had been a few rooms away or something, I would have needed a steadying hand by my side.

I didn't feel tired or particularly open to sharing my inner conversations, but I wasn't relaxing. I was very aware of my external environment: the guides, the lovely art, and the comfortable blankets. My guide sensed I needed a booster dose, and I agreed. I wanted to get to a mental place where I could relax into the MDMA and trust my guides. It was like how I knew when I needed another cup of green tea for a caffeine boost to push through a work project.

After taking the booster dose, I cuddled up under some blankets with my super soft, 1980s-like bulky socks and my plush eye mask. My guides asked me to listen to what the medicine wanted to tell me.

Unfortunately, I couldn't quiet myself.

So instead of lying down quietly, I took off my eye mask and engaged my guide and therapist. I think my brain thought, "Hey, if I keep them occupied, they won't focus on me." Brilliant right?

My guide mirrored back to me what I wanted to talk about. He didn't direct the conversation. He simply held space in the room for me to direct the journey. He gently nudged against anything unhealthy that he heard from me, though. For instance, he quickly realized that I didn't think I was allowed to take up space in this world. I felt it was a mistake I even existed. I had a target on my back because the universe knew it had made a mistake. After mirroring my conversation to clarify what I was saying, he explained a simple concept.

The sun is the sun.

The sun provided warmth and nourished people. But the sun never stopped being the sun even if people got sunburnt, chose to put on sunscreen, or went indoors.

The sun is the sun. It belongs where it is.

Jill is Jill. She belongs where she is.

The conversation was so powerful that it was one of my only real memories of the day.

My guide was trying to break through all the noise in my head and used the third person when he said, "Jill is a person who is Jill. She can be in her fullness. She deserves to live."

It sounded great.

I didn't believe it.

I explained why I didn't believe it. My father didn't care who or what I was. I tried to explain a few different ways that he would hurt me no matter what. My guides didn't disagree or say any of the polite things people say about family. I had heard society's message, *family forgives family*, my entire life. But here, in this room, my guides didn't try to whitewash any of my feelings.

They held the space in the journey room safe for me to express my fears, and when I settled, they encouraged me to put my eye mask back on and try to work with the medicine. When I did, MDMA kept my internal conversations flowing.

I later learned that guarded people have a standard way of dealing with a first journey. In hindsight, I now understand that while I trusted my guides, my traumatized inner children did not. They knew that throughout my life, no adult ever helped me get away from my father.

It was several months and a tech glitch or two before I got the day's recording. I quickly time-stamped and transcribed my first journey into thirty written pages. The following segments showed my five-year-old inner child's hissy fit from that day. She just stopped my brain from working when she didn't like the direction of the conversations.

Jill: I have never been permitted to be who I want to be.
Guide: Who would need to give you permission?
Jill: The universe. The universe.
Guide: So maybe you want to go inside and ask the universe that same question. Who would need to give you permission? What is the universe's answer to you?

Jill: It stopped talking.

———————

Guide: Same question. Who would permit you to be who you want to be?
Jill: The universe. The universe would let me be me and not smack me down.
Guide: Ask the universe again. See what it says.
Jill: Ask the universe what? How quickly are you going to smack me down?
Guide: No, what would permit me to be what I want to be? You kind of feel like something out there is not permitting you. I am asking you to fact-check that.
Jill: We need to revisit that because it is not coming easily.

———————

These segments illustrate my deep-seated fear of practically everything. When my brain wouldn't give me the answers, I stopped talking. Then, when I started talking again, I shifted topics.

———————

Guide: See what shows up in the quiet.
Jill: I am not good at that.
Guide: Discover that. Discover the edge of quiet. What is it like being quiet?
Jill: I am terrible at it. There is always activity. There is always motion. I always have to stay one step ahead. I have to anticipate. I have to stay one step ahead. I gotta keep preparing. That is why I am not quiet.

Therapist: It is not safe.
Jill: Things can sneak up on me when it is quiet. If I'm not paying attention, shit comes at me out of nowhere.
Guide: It must be exhausting. Is it?

———————

Guide: What is Jill desiring now? What do you want now?
Jill: I want love, and I want fun, and I want not to be working so hard. I have worked my ass off with a constant fear that it can all be taken away.
Guide: Is it the working hard or the fear that makes it hard?
Jill: The pace.
Guide: Right, but what is driving the pace?
Jill: The fear.
Guide: So, we are back at fear.

———————

At around the fifth hour after ingesting MDMA, I quickly "snapped out" of my enhanced state, which ended the journey. I still had the medicine in my system, but I wouldn't let it do any more searching through my memories. I shut the journey down, and to me, it seemed only to have lasted about forty-five minutes. My guide mentioned I was almost textbook guarded, and that the suddenness of getting out of the journey was a signal of someone with lots of work to do. I remember winking with pride to my therapist a few moments after I snapped out of it. I had control back. My conscious mind was in the driver's seat.

It was like I had woken up from sleep instantly alert on a

weekday because of my internal clock versus a weekend morning of being lazy and taking my time to get out of bed. I'm not sure why I was so proud of myself, but that was the feeling. I knew they hadn't "gotten" me, and I was still safe.

Being endlessly curious, I asked how my guide had determined I was guarded. He gave me a party analogy that made me seem like the rudest host ever! It was like I had invited them to a party during the journey, but I simply wouldn't open the door when they got to my house. All the windows were locked too. I didn't make the party quiet—they knew there was a party—they were just stuck on the porch.

I didn't quite understand how I had distanced my guides from my subconscious, but I was impressed with myself. I had managed to protect myself, even medicated. That was a metric that proved the strength of my inner children who had kept me safe my entire life.

The process of returning to the present consisted of eating some food and drinking water in the sitting area on the other side of the room. We then had a lovely grounding walk outside. As I let the grass tickle my feet, my pride soon turned to embarrassment that I had wasted their time. I was disappointed that all the time invested in my talk therapy sessions and the entire day for this first journey seemed to be for nothing. I hung back while we walked because the thrill of having control back gave me a shameful pink flush. But they waited for me and eased my concerns. They assured me that work had been done and asked me to be kind to myself in the coming days. They explained the depth of my trauma and my mental protections had years of practice, so that healing would take time. That explanation made sense to me. After all, if my fears and extreme physical responses were easily healed, I think I would have successfully gotten rid of them decades before.

After the walk, I remember getting right back into Type A Jill who always had to get stuff done. I helped by tidying up the journey room. I folded my blanket and cleaned up our little food containers. I look back now, and I realize I did everything I could to regain my independence and not rely on my guides' help any longer.

It doesn't feel great admitting I shut out my guides. But if I am going to stay as true to the story as possible, then the reality of my brain stopping me from healing needs to be normalized. My inner children didn't have any trust that things could get better. They didn't have any reason to believe adults would help. I also wondered if my inner five-year-old had used the day to test my guides. Were they going to give up and be as useless to me as every other adult when I was a child?

I figured this was another failed attempt to find mental peace. With my bag under my arm, I waited for my ride. Since I didn't remember most of the last five hours, I felt like a failure. After Carl's death, I tried a six-week meditation program, boot camped hard until I screwed up my shoulder, and even tried a year on the anti-depressant Wellbutrin. None of those solutions had any lasting impact on my happiness, and I figured I would add this experience to the *Shit That Didn't Work* list.

As I walked out of the room into the fall Pennsylvania air, I tried not to cry as I figured the day had been a waste of time.

Chapter 10

Quick Shit

When my boyfriend picked me up, he let me sit and rest while he drove. In about two minutes into the drive, I heard my inner voice start to chat with me. Until this MDMA journey, I had never listened to my inner voice before. While I was a classic "closed off" patient during the journey, I learned quickly that the time was not wasted. I'm sure my inner voice was itching to say *bless her heart,* but instead kindly chatted with me to change my perspective about something I had always *known.* Below is how my mind changed from *knowing* I was an inconvenience to people to understanding that my friends would readily lend a hand if I asked.

> **Jill:** I hate being an inconvenience. My boyfriend had to drop me off and pick me up. I hate asking for help.
> **Inner Voice**: Why?
> **Jill**: Because I was an inconvenience. I was constantly shuffled. There was never enough money. I never felt either parent had any genuine interest in me as a person.

I immediately learned that the medicine used my memories to explain my inner conversations. The same way I could get a great idea during an exercise class or while singing in the shower—that's how my memories worked. They just appeared in my mind without my body reacting in fear or sadness. Sometimes it felt like the memories *floated* into focus, too. They got sharper and more precise when I focused on them.

●●●●●●●

The first memory was when I was between eight and ten years old. My father had custody of me, and I saw my mother every other weekend. The memory that surfaced was the weekend routine of first going to the mall and getting something crafty at the toy store. I would sit in my mother's apartment on Saturday afternoons and Sunday mornings, working on a craft kit, and watching old movies. I knew she was getting high because of the smoke that escaped from under the closed bedroom door. We maybe spent an hour together during those weekends.

Then the memory of my father surfaced when I was seventeen. My father would "forget" to pick me up from work and assume I would find a ride home. It was too much for him to get up from watching TV and eating ice cream straight from the container to pick me up from my after-school job. This was before cell phones and Uber. It would have been so much easier to know he wouldn't be picking me up, but he never gave me a heads up that he wouldn't be there. He made it clear it was an inconvenience for him as he chose to wave me

**off from his chair when I managed to get home.
I didn't have the luxury of showing any anger,
so I always just went to my room.**

●●●●●●●

After these memories faded, I had this internal
conversation:

> **Inner Voice:** Are you an inconvenience right now?
> **Jill:** No, this was just a drop-off and pick-up. No
> big deal at all. Only a quick ride. This man loves
> me. This is not even a thing on a potential list of
> inconveniences.
> **Inner Voice:** Have you been an inconvenience?
> **Jill:** No, not really. After the age of twenty-five, the
> people in my life, for the most part, tried to help me
> in my career. People have been kind. Even when I
> was hospitalized and asked for help, it was given
> with such warmth and kindness. People liked being
> able to help.
> **Inner Voice:** Why do you think you are an
> inconvenience to people?
> **Jill:** (Looking out the car's side window because of
> tears.) My parents didn't have time for me as a
> child. After my mom shot herself, I lived with a
> series of relatives until my father could take me
> years later. I was always the new kid in school and
> the extra bed in a bedroom. I tried my best always
> to fit in and not cause any trouble. My father once
> blamed me for his live-in girlfriend leaving him,
> and my mother blamed me for her breakdown when
> my father came back into my life.

RESCUING JILL

I wasn't an inconvenience to them.
I was a handy scapegoat.
Inner Voice: Don't you have friends who offer to help you when you need them?
Jill: Yes.
Inner Voice: Occasionally asking for a favor from friends doesn't make you, as a person, an inconvenience. Let's stop thinking that way and let people help you.

The conversation happened this clearly, in the car, on the way home. It set the stage for how the flurry of conversations happened over the next few days, weeks, and even months. My perspectives, beliefs, assumptions, and absolutes were no longer absolutes at all.

I captured these kinds of internal conversations because my guides strongly suggested that I journal. They said integration phases are rich with perspective shifts. While I didn't understand how the integration phase worked, my therapist had told me it was 40% of the process, so I took it very seriously. I made sure to journal daily and sometimes went back to the keyboard two or three times when my mind was particularly active. I wanted to capture as much as possible because they said my mind might work fast, and some small perspective shifts might zoom in and out of focus quickly. Interestingly, they mentioned that patients sometimes lose track of how they thought about their lives before their MDMA journey.

I didn't believe them initially, but boy—they were right.

Yet again, my guides gave me great advice. When I look at my journals now, I'm surprised that some of the things I *knew* were real— weren't.

Chapter 11

Integration Understood

I went on my first journey without any clear understanding of how the integration phase of my treatment would work. I remember my guides emphasized journaling and giving my mind the grace it needed to think and explore what came to mind.

Since my first journey was on a Thursday, I lounged around the house on Friday. The MDMA hangover took my energy, and I couldn't get rid of an annoying headache. I nursed it by eating well and sipping water and tea throughout the day.

I also thought a lot about that first conversation with my inner voice when my boyfriend drove me home the day before. Since my guides knew I had heard a strong, female voice in my head during the journey, and they hadn't sounded any alarms, I figured I didn't hear the voices in a "she needs to be committed" kind of way. I wasn't scared of this voice one bit. While it was new, it felt oddly *right*. It was like a puzzle piece that doesn't look like it could possibly fit, but suddenly pops into place. I finally didn't feel alone at my core.

I learned that my first experience in the car was the exact same footprint that my integration would follow through my healing. If I had a thought or emotion that somehow tied to my intentions, then specific childhood memories would come into focus without my body feeling the fear or anger those memories usually created. I might also have a conversation with my inner voice. Sometimes I had a combination of an old memory and internal dialogue. Reviewing my memories from my adult perspective allowed me to shift my feelings about those memories. It was like when I was terrified watching *Poltergeist* so many years ago, but I can laugh at the special effects now.

But I had to be willing to dive into the pain of those emotions.

It felt like my brain was finally free to start rethinking my past that first weekend. The MDMA seemed to have ripped open a bag of Pop Rocks in my brain because I had a flurry of ideas and memories coming at me! I felt an energy inside me that I couldn't remember feeling before. It spurred countless hours of journal writing with tiny, slight perspective shifts and many unanswered questions.

When I talked to my therapist at our scheduled check-in (we talked every two weeks, whenever schedules allowed, for our regular talk therapy sessions), I remember using way too many jazz hands to explain how excited I was at the spark and sizzle in my brain! When we chatted and I wrote in my journals, I attributed the process to *the medicine*. It is important to note that I meant while the MDMA was in my system only during the journey. For me, it seemed that during the journey, the MDMA had highlighted relevant memories deep in my subconscious. The same way I highlight specific lines in a book to refer to later, the MDMA found the memories that somehow tied back to my intentions and highlighted those suckers bright yellow for future reference!

I wish I could explain why specific memories were highlighted or how the order in which I dealt with particular memories was determined. Looking at my life differently was not a linear process. My healing didn't start at age five and work forward or start at fifty and work backward. I would make perspective shifts throughout the healing, only to sometimes find I needed more healing to shift a perspective entirely. Almost every time I thought differently about my father, I thought I was done. Then I would be disappointed when another memory would surface.

I had layers and layers of trauma tied to my father. Consequently, memories about him are in each of the journeys. Just like a relay runner, I had to get around the track of my trauma enough to pass along the baton to another layer of trauma to heal.

Since I couldn't explain the direction my healing went, I simply pointed to the medicine during the process. I figured the medicine drew me to specific memories because those were the memories where I had trapped emotions from the trauma *at the time of the memories.*

So, when I attribute to the medicine a fuzzy memory coming into focus, I'm referring to MDMA's work from my journey. After all, without MDMA exploring my brain, letting me be more empathetic to myself, and dulling my physical responses to horrific memories, I never would have revisited my childhood in such detail.

Chapter 12

Dog Walking

Between Sadie's hectic schedule of eating, sleeping, and protecting the house from some sketchy squirrels, she gets a few walks a day. She is always down for a treat and runs to the door when I pick up her red leash. We routinely wander around my development, which is full of trees and lots of good doggie smells. I didn't realize, until my journeys, how much I let my mind relax during those walks. All those sayings that being in nature is good for us—turns out that shit is true.

I didn't know walking Sadie was my form of meditation. I've never been very good at traditional meditation because I couldn't slow down my mind. Even when my adult life was perfectly safe, my inner self was always looking over my shoulder. In my head, I always had a guard on red alert!

That Friday afternoon, we meandered around the development during her dog walk. I was surprised to hear that inner female voice, to whom I had just been introduced, start chatting with me. As Sadie and I rounded the top of the hill, I heard, "What could my parents' lives have been like growing up? What led them to be such unhappy adults?"

One of the studied effects of MDMA is compassion, but I had no idea I would start to look at my parents in a new, compassionate way.

These were utterly new questions for me. Remember how surprised I was looking at my parent's wedding album and not seeing any joy? I didn't think about my parents' lives before I was born. My parents didn't talk about their childhoods. The only grandparent I remember is my father's mother. I never noticed the red flags that neither parent spoke about their parents. In fact, I only knew that my parents grew up in Philadelphia, but I didn't know where.

Just like I remembered memories of my childhood on the way home from the journey, that's precisely how integration made me realize how my childhood memories shaped me. The medicine brought me two dusty memories that seemed to float into focus from wherever they lived in my head for over thirty years.

●●●●●●●

First, when I was seventeen, I visited my father's mother. We sat at her dining room table and finished breakfast in one of the many pink condos. I remember trying to answer her question about why I had lived with my mother from age ten to sixteen.

I tried to explain how my father had beaten me and had thrown me out of his house when I was ten. I remember she looked away and waved me off with a sweep of her arm. I distinctly remember her paper-thin, sun-spotted hands that signaled for me to stop talking. She didn't want to hear any of it. There was an awkward silence as we sat at the old 1970s green, vinyl-covered table. I stared at her and re-learned that my history wasn't important to any adult. I felt isolated, and that

feeling sculpted my internal dialog that what happened in my childhood was shameful, was never discussed, and most importantly, seemingly deserved. There would be no questioning her son's behavior in front of me—ever.

I never learned their dynamic and why my father was allowed to treat everyone in his path so terribly. His life was a series of failed relationships and jobs. For the first time in my life, I wondered if he was abused as a child and if my grandmother felt guilty? Or was my grandmother wholly tuned out and unable to really see the child she raised?

●●●●●●●

That memory faded, and by this time in our walk, Sadie and I were at the bottom of my development's hill. We walked over to the picnic table near the creek. As I looked at the water, the second memory that came into focus was my mother when she tried to leave my father in the early 1970s.

●●●●●●●

My mother told me that our very Jewish, patriarchal relatives weren't supportive, and each would only take us in for a few days. Suddenly it occurred to me that she never told me much about those years except for one

57

story. While I remembered the story my mother always described, I realized something was *off*.

My mother told me that when we went to "one of the aunts," *I* got "us" in trouble because *I* opened the refrigerator to get something to eat. I had to be younger than five, so I'm sure I carefully hatched a super-secret scheme to eat something. I'm guessing I tried to open the door with my toddler strength and got caught red-handed! I don't have any memory of this story, so I've always depended on my mother's unfinished version.

That was it. She never told me who those relatives were, how long we stayed with them, and why they didn't help. She only told me that one refrigerator story—repeatedly. I even remember she retold that story when I was in her apartment before she died. So, I heard that story even until my early forties. I always thought that story was supposed to show how heartless our relatives were. Not only wouldn't they take us in, but they also wouldn't feed a child.

●●●●●●●

Now, sitting on that picnic bench while Sadie did her sniffing thing in the grass, I realized that the story was a little weird. She never explained how many people she had asked for help. I never got a list of relatives. She never mentioned why *all* those other people wouldn't let her stay with them. The only story about why we couldn't get any help to leave my father was about me "stealing" food.

I never put together that she didn't talk about those family members. Instead, I internalized that I was a burden that prevented my mother from getting away from her abusive marriage.

Maybe the MDMA was letting me be a bit more compassionate to myself?

It was much more likely my mother used me as a handy scapegoat to explain why we couldn't leave my father for good.

Just one day into my integration, I realized that a toddler trying to get a snack wasn't a logical reason for my mother's family not to help. Maybe she didn't have family, or maybe my mother was always too needy for our relatives like I remembered her behavior with me? For the first time, I realized I didn't know anything about my mother's family, and I couldn't trust the one story she had told me my whole life. My mother had passed away years before, so I couldn't ask her any of my new questions.

As Sadie and I walked home, I realized I didn't know much about my parents' lives. I had heard occasional stories about my mother's father, the gambler, but other than that, I couldn't remember any childhood stories from either of them. How did I not realize that was a huge red flag?

I did now.

I understood my parents had their whole lives behind them when I was born, and since they didn't talk about happy childhood memories, I have to assume there weren't many.

The integration had me thinking about my parents as

people with lives before my birth for the first time. I realized they probably both had less than ideal childhoods. This didn't change how I felt about them and their parenting mistakes. It allowed me to empathize with them. It was the start of me allowing them the grace to be flawed people, doing the best they could with what preparation they had in their lives to be adults.

In my journals, I wrote about the nuance of this therapy. For the first time, I looked at my parents from an adult's perspective and realized that they were hurting in their ways before I ever came along.

*Astute readers might have noticed that my mind was working on the perspective shifts around my parents, which did not extend to my grandmother. That memory of her at the table waving me off stayed ingrained, with the *adults don't help* interpretation until well after my third journey. I mention it now because it illustrates the layers of trauma. My grandmother's feeble response was just filed in my mind as proof that adults didn't help and didn't become a specific trauma point. Only much, much later in my treatment, in my fourth therapeutic journey, did I start to empathize with what she may have been facing.

Chapter 13

Mental Folders

By Sunday of that weekend, I had journaled like crazy. The journals were full of questions as I looked at dusty childhood memories. I think the MDMA jostled my understanding of the world a bit, and my journals from that first weekend rambled with my newfound curiosity about my history.

Through all the memories, though, I kept circling one in particular. My journals showed me I had a ton of trapped emotions from getting kicked out of my mother's apartment when I was sixteen.

That memory was so putrid; I thought I had filed it in my brain's "Life Sucks and is Unpredictable" folder. Unfortunately, it was one of many childhood memories in that folder. But I realized by Sunday that my brain also had a folder called "Jill Fucked Up Big Time." This memory of when I was sixteen was the only one stored there.

●●●●●●●

When I was sixteen, my world turned upside down. I always remembered it as my mother throwing me out of her apartment, and I had to live the rest of my high school career in another state with my abusive father.

I didn't have contact with my father from ages ten to sixteen because I lived with my mother during those years. He threw me out of his house when I was ten. Then at sixteen, after six years of no contact, he came into my life on weekends and flashed money around like it grew on trees. He took me out to eat and bought me clothes. He was nice to me.

My mother and I didn't have much money, so I was enthralled with new clothes and music. He appeared kind and fatherly. He made me forget what it had been like living with him years ago. I wanted a father. I wanted attention. Looking back, though, I know his presence in our lives pushed my mother further into her depression and fear. I was too busy being a teenager with good grades, potential scholarships, and great friends. Back then, I had hope for a future. I was so wrapped up in being a teenager that I didn't see any red flags with my mother's behavior. She came home from work and went to her bedroom and got high like always.

I thought my father had changed, and I could have both parents in my life. I accepted his gifts and started to trust him again. In the most child-centric way, I thought I was a good enough daughter that I could get to have both parents in my life.

One afternoon, in my mother's apartment, it was me, my mother, and my father. I can't remember why we were together. But I remember my mother's eyes were wide with fear, and she slapped me. I hate that her face is still burned in my memory because I think she hated me at that moment. She ordered me to leave. I've come to believe she was desperate to get my father out of her life, which meant getting me out of her life. Within ten minutes, I had to live with my father in another state. I was devastated to leave my friends and uproot my life in my junior year of high school. Before I had lived with my mother, I hadn't been in a school system for an entire year.

Most importantly, the shiny veneer of my father's kindness and wealth disappeared in the car ride to his apartment. His verbal abuse started quickly, and for the entire ride, I heard that I was stupid and a troublemaker. I got quiet and tried to disappear into the passenger seat. When we got to his one-bedroom apartment, which was hoarder-littered with newspapers and a few odd pieces of furniture, I knew the rest of my high school career would be tinged with trying to stay safe from my father. Unlike when I was young, my mother wasn't a buffer anymore.

I was sad and angry. I was sad that, yet again, my parents had done stupid shit that affected me. But I was also steaming angry at myself. I had trusted my father. I had let him back into my life. It was my fault that everything I had worked for academically crumbled, and I couldn't fix it. My junior class rank plummeted from 8th to 54th when I enrolled at my new school. That school move killed several scholarship opportunities. I had seen academics as a way out of my life that had been littered with abuse, poverty, drugs, and suicides. To me, losing that one lifeline knocked my ego down quite a few pegs. I was embarrassed that my path to get out evaporated because I trusted my father. I remember losing my belief in hope during that time. Hope was what other people had.

●●●●●●●

I internalized from that point forward that my decision-making sucked, and I knew that my decision-making sucked for the next thirty years of my life. Trusting my father and allowing him in my life was *my* wrong decision. I never saw that I had no control over my father and that he was an adult. The trapped emotions from this age were me thinking that I *allowed* my father back into my life and that it *proved* I made terrible decisions. That's why the folder "Jill Fucked Up Big Time" existed in my brain.

One transcript from the first journey made it clear how this trauma point stayed embedded in my mind:

———————

Jill: And just to let you know that I am deeply embarrassed that we are still talking about issues from being sixteen.

Guide: I don't think you have issues with being sixteen.

Jill: Then I am not explaining myself well enough.

Guide: I think it is more like sixteen feels like a safe place to stop.

Jill: What do you mean?

Guide: Well, you want to remember sixteen everything getting dashed. What was the conversation you were having about yourself?

Jill: I failed. I didn't manipulate my mother and father just long enough to get what I needed.

Guide: That is interesting. "I didn't manipulate long enough to get what I needed. So, I failed."

Jill: I failed. I allowed my father back into my life.

Because of the trauma I felt over the decision to trust my father, I figured out that I constantly questioned every crucial decision for the rest of my life. From that sixteen-year-old's perspective, I didn't have good decision-making skills. I made the mother of all bad choices by allowing my father in my life. I didn't consider my mother's fear. Those child-centric feelings that *my* decision had *destroyed* my chances to get away from my parents and the poverty in which they lived stayed trapped within me. I mean, I knew my parents were inept. I *should* have known just how incompetent back then and made better decisions.

Trauma is deeply personal. This shame (that my decision-making skills were crap and I deserved what I got having to live with my father) was an undercurrent my entire life. If I had shared with my friends, they would have said, "No. You were sixteen, and your parents should have acted as caring adults." But even if I had trusted someone with my shame, I wouldn't have believed the obvious. That trauma was stuck at age sixteen, and the only thing I knew at age sixteen was that I fucked up big time.

So it was a surprise that just four days after my first journey, I started to attack the shame around this part of my life in my journal. I mean, this shame was deeply buried. I hadn't talked about it in over twenty-five years.

> *Why did my father come back into my life so hard at sixteen? Why was it so crucial for him to have my attention that he threw money around he didn't have? Did he want to fuck up my future, or was he lonely? What did he want from a sixteen-year-old?*

Suddenly I found I could write about this time of my life without my stomach getting queasy or my shoulders crunching up to my ears. It was like I was *looking* at the memory more than *feeling* the anger and shame of that memory. I wrote in my journal:

> *I am coming more and more to conclude that my father's decisions were all about him, and I won't ever know why. I think I was very little in the equations, which means a lot. That means the universe wasn't after me then. He was doing whatever in his warped mind he wanted to do. He has always lacked empathy.*

Just days into my integration, I started to see my father's behavior as *his* in response to his own needs. I had never looked at that time in my life that way. I had internalized that I somehow deserved everything terrible that had happened to me.

This realization was huge! This was tectonic plates shifting huge! After thinking a specific way about that time in my life, for my entire life, I started to look at that time with different eyes within days of my first journey. I looked at that time from an adult perspective. Those trapped emotions were from when I was sixteen, with only a sixteen-year-old's perspective. Looking at the memories from an adult's perspective was suddenly possible.

I felt lighter. Starting to lose the shame was like taking off a layer when I came in from the cold. I began to understand that my father would create chaos to satisfy his needs no matter what. It didn't matter how old I was or my needs. My father operated for his satisfaction more than anything else.

There were dozens of similar entries in my journal over the next few weeks. I tried to unravel my trapped emotions from the eighteen months I lived with him. There was a lot to unpack from the second half of my junior year to my first year in college.

When I thought back to my intentions for the journey, it suddenly made sense why I was so afraid of the future. How would I craft a promising future if I thought I couldn't make good decisions? My trapped emotions from age sixteen overshadowed a lifetime of excellent choices. I lived through trauma-tinged glasses since my inner sixteen-year-old couldn't see any of the fantastic decisions I made as an adult.

Chapter 14

"Jill is Alone" Folder

As I entered the second week after the journey, I couldn't hear too much from my inner voice. Even when Sadie and I walked, I couldn't hear any chatter. I think it was because I didn't understand how to use the integration process well. Because of my journaling, I know I didn't trust that my mind could change so much because I wasn't getting notable perspective shifts every day like I did that first weekend. It wasn't until I went back to my journals with a more precise eye that I saw the healing trends as the integration unfolded. But when I wrote those journal entries, I was too close to the slight shifts to see the big picture of my healing.

I wrote about the beginning of my integration and compared it to a beautiful campfire that sparked and sizzled. That fire had turned into a black pile of cold ash. I wasn't getting zippy perspective shifts anymore.

I wrote that I missed my inner voice. I had pushed that inner voice and intuition so deep inside me for my whole life that silence was my status quo state. I reverted to how I knew to live before my MDMA journey.

Because I missed my internal voice so much, I started to look at more traditional ways of meditation than walking Sadie. I repeatedly tried to sit and follow my breath, but I was a solid D- meditation student because my thoughts rambled. After trying a few phone meditation apps, I turned to YouTube and tried some guided meditations. I finally lucked out with an Internal Family Systems meditation focused on "the self." I had stumbled across Internal Family Systems (IFS) via Instagram and found that picturing some of my anxieties/issues as "parts" of me was helpful. For instance, I visualized two parts: a super tall warrior female who was always ready for battle, and a workaholic stuck on a treadmill that could not stop. The guided meditation let me visit with my "parts" and then let me walk away from them. I felt relaxed after this meditation and used it a few times a week.

I improved from a D- to a C+ with this meditation practice. It didn't matter what my imagination dreamed up during my meditations because my mind was focused on me separating from so many trauma symptoms (overwork) and fears (needing a warrior on standby). This technique was great practice for seeing my thoughts and fears without feeling the PTSD physical symptoms.

But I still didn't hear my inner voice.

Instead, I became increasingly aware of uncomfortable feelings.

I was even more disappointed in the small amount of work I felt I had done during my first journey. I hadn't expected unpleasant feelings to be part of the integration process. I misunderstood and thought I was at the end of the last 40% of the process my therapist described. I didn't realize she had used those percentages to describe each journey cycle.

The most upsetting feeling was my sense of isolation that I couldn't put back into the "Jill is Alone" folder in my head during that time. That folder usually flipped open around the holidays because there wasn't a lot of family on my mother's side. When I left my father at nineteen, I became the family's outcast because I refused to put up with the family's bullshit narrative that he was allowed to treat me however he wanted without consequences.

That folder was like an overstuffed suitcase that I couldn't close.

At the beginning of the second week of integration, I felt profoundly alone. I wrote paragraph after paragraph of how much I missed Carl until I concluded, sadly:

> *I was worth something to Carl. He was it. I wasn't worth anything to anyone else.*

That was the first time my journals started to touch on my sense of worthlessness. My isolation wasn't just that I didn't have people in my life. Those intense feelings of isolation also stemmed from not feeling I was worth having people in my life.

Chapter 15

Jill is Mean

I continued to explore my sense of isolation in my journals but took an odd detour into a work thing that threaded its way through many journal entries. I think most work things in big corporations are exceptionally dull, so I won't go into details that don't matter here. What mattered was that I journaled about how razor-thin the wall between my politeness and my meanness was getting over this work thing. I wrote pages and pages where I attempted to release all my snark and venom through my journaling to remain professional at work.

Finally, I had enough of one coworker's shenanigans.

When politeness stopped working, I sent an eviscerating email. Everyone who has used email at work can identify snarkiness through professional wording about impact and corporate metrics like KPIs. I made it clear, with attached email threads, that I was done playing, and one of my coworkers had to step up or step aside.

I felt queasy about sending that email because I included leadership folks on the CC line, and everyone could see my *meanness*.

In general, I detested confrontation and had worked hard to avoid it. I had learned incredibly early in life that fewer beatings happened when I didn't stand up for myself. But that email was necessary, appropriate, and resulted in required changes. Unfortunately, reality didn't matter to my body, and I felt queasy for days after hitting the send button. I felt vulnerable because now the one secret I worked most to hide was out. I was fundamentally a mean person. I had placed a target on my back by showing I was mean. Now people would be out to get me.

I didn't know how I knew that people would brand me *mean* and what harmful retribution there would be. My body just *knew* my meanness was a problem.

The worst part was how terrible I felt about having to bust out Snarky Jill. This situation was resolved after my email, and all I had done was assert myself. But to me, I had shown my cards that I can be professionally assertive with an unmistakable bite.

Part of me knew I was overreacting. Just like the initial panic attack, I knew my thinking was a bit over the top, but darned if I could stop feeling in danger because I was *mean* for sending that thoroughly researched, clarifying email that produced results.

Within a few days of stepping back from my emotions and trying to sort them out, the dusty memory of my father clawing up the steps to grab my leg, drag me down the stairs, and throw me against the wall floated into focus. That was the memory that Kathy and I had worked on with EMDR (eye movement desensitization and reprocessing treatment). I no longer had the dreaded stomach-dropping fear when I remembered my father's raging scowl as he climbed up the stairs like a charging bull elephant. But I was surprised that this memory held a deeper level of trauma. I journaled:

●●●●●●●

The first time I felt profoundly alone was when I was maybe four, and my father grabbed me at the top of the stairs by my right leg, dragged me down

the stairs, and threw me into a wall before going back upstairs to beat my mother. With the side of my head hurting, I huddled up, clutched my Dressy Betsy doll, and heard my mother's screams.

I didn't even try to help her.

● ● ● ● ● ● ●

My journals now had a weird mix of fear, isolation, and meanness. It made sense that I was scared of hearing my mother getting beaten. It made sense that I felt isolated because no one ever came to help us when my father's fits of rage went unchecked.

The last line from my memory, *"I didn't even try to help her"* made me gasp.

Who wouldn't help another person? Well, someone who was fundamentally mean, right?

When I looked at the journals, I teared up. In trying to be small and protect myself, I thought I was the meanest person ever because I didn't help my mother. That was my proof that I was rotten to the core *mean*.

I didn't run up those steps to help.

I didn't run out the door to get a neighbor.

I didn't shriek in any attempt to pull my father's attention away from battering her.

I had lived my entire life *knowing* I was a cold-hearted little girl.

Of course, I wasn't worth loving. Why would my mother love a little girl who didn't help her?

While I journaled about this incident after my first journey, it took many months for me to share with my guides this work thing that allowed this deeply embedded shame to show itself to me. In my case, I could only deal with issues I could admit to and talk about. I wouldn't go near this deep shame about who I was at my core until my third journey. I mention my shame here because this was the actual timeline. But trauma healing for me was not linear.

I hid my shame for months. I was scared my guides might dump me if they knew how *mean* I was and that I was not worth their time and effort.

Chapter 16

Mom Tried to Escape

My journals about feeling alone also touched on my mother's attempt to kill herself with a shotgun. I was five, and my mother had already tried a few times to leave this world via pills and razor blades. Her arms had the unsuccessful, crisscrossed scars that she explained away with a fictitious car accident.

●●●●●●●●

My father and I came home and found my mother in the upstairs bathroom. I remember her on the floor with blood across her stomach. But the sense of being alone hit hard when I watched the ambulance's red and blue lights swirl from my neighbor's door. I remember being alone and scared for my mommy. I don't know how long I stood at that door or what happened after that ambulance left. My body remembered how alone and out of place I felt standing there.

I felt like the last kid at a party after all the other kids had been picked up and the parents were putting away the decorations.

I didn't have anywhere to go.

●●●●●●●●

I look back now, and I think my five-year-old brain was

overloaded with everything I didn't understand.

I knew life was tough and lonely. That much I knew.

While walking Sadie one afternoon, I suddenly looked at my mother's shotgun suicide attempt differently. I had always harbored a bit of resentment that she was willing to leave me with my father, so I hadn't spent much time in my adulthood thinking about her suicide attempts.

I don't know what made me think about hunting as we walked by the creek. Maybe the geese and ducks that waddled into the water turned a few gears in my head as we approached. Suddenly I realized that my father was the hunter in the family, and he was the owner of the shotgun my mother used.

My mother didn't own a gun.

My mother didn't know how to handle a gun. She didn't know how to load a gun. Heck, she couldn't even kill herself with one.

It was like a forehead slap when I realized that my father had made his loaded shotgun available to a woman with numerous suicide attempts under her belt. A long-lost memory of my mother telling me the gun had been kept in their bedroom floated into focus.

The medicine let me empathize with my mother in a unique way now. My mother wasn't trying to leave me. My mother was trying to escape my father. The nuclear option of shooting herself became her only option. Her initial cries for help with pills and razor blades had been ignored. I'm sure she, and he, thought a shotgun was a sure thing. Later that day I wrote in my journal:

I guess he got tired of her fucking it up.

Chapter 17

Belonging

Being an only child with very little family, I always felt sad around holidays. I didn't have the love and warmth from a family that I saw on TV sitcoms during their holiday-themed shows.

I was accustomed to feeling a little low and even a bit jealous of people with family during the holidays. But my holidays with Carl had been wonderful, and I had recently started to take back the holidays by spending them doing whatever I wanted to do. If making the holidays *mine* meant binging Netflix and eating ice cream for breakfast, then that's what it meant.

So, it was a little surprising that my integration had me feeling *holiday lonely* when there wasn't a holiday looming on the calendar. Plus, I had been making my holidays a lot more fun by permitting myself to do whatever the fuck I wanted to do.

My writing in several journals touched on when I was five to eight years old and living with a few relatives. After my mother had shot herself and needed to recuperate, I was immediately shuffled to my grandmother and then to a few aunts. I remembered the feeling of being the new kid in school, the kid who didn't have nice clothes, the kid who bunked with cousins, and the kid who did her best to stay quiet and not draw attention to herself. I didn't make many friends because I was enrolled in schools for only months at a time. The first time I was in a school for an entire year was seventh grade.

Belonging

I never felt I belonged, and I never felt I had a *home*. I lived in many places as a child, but the childhood house I remembered at Lanner Street until I was five was full of violence, pain, and fear.

No place I ever lived, with either parent, ever had the warmth of a *home*.

I looked over those journals and tried to figure out how they fit with the sense of isolation I was feeling now. I thought my memories showed why I never felt I belonged anywhere, and looking at my early history, that made more sense than ever. Maybe I wasn't alone as much as I didn't feel like I belonged?

There was something bigger at play here, though. This wasn't the normal *I don't have family, and the holidays aren't fun* feeling. I felt this isolation like a heavy stone in my stomach. My body was telling me I was destined to be alone.

What was weird was that I didn't even feel like I belonged in my own house where I had lived for twenty years. I felt displaced and isolated in a warm and lovely home I had built with Carl and didn't know why.

I wrote quite a few times that I felt I would *always* be alone too. I noted how often I wrote about my sense of isolation through blurry tears in my journals. My loneliness seemed to spread from my belly and become woven into the very fabric of who I was. I concluded a few times that I didn't *deserve* to be anything but alone.

One poignant memory that floated into focus at this point was a work trip to NY. I had always thought the negative feelings about this memory were about money. It took me a few passes before I figured out this memory was about feeling like I didn't *belong* and would never *fit in* with groups of women with children and family.

●●●●●●●●

A few years ago, I had been in New York for a work-sponsored women's conference, and I thought I was super excited to go shopping in stores that wouldn't dream of having locations in my boring suburbs. I ditched my fellow conference gals before the evening meal and went wandering. Yet, when I got to the stores, I felt like a fish out of water. I had this intense, full-body flush of not being good enough, not having enough money, and I didn't find anything interesting because "It isn't like you could afford it anyway. Stop embarrassing yourself."

When I stopped and had dinner at an adorable Spanish restaurant, I wondered why I had this emotional reaction to shopping. I had plenty of shopping money. As I sat comfortably alone at the bustling restaurant's bar, listening to the lively chatter around me, I realized that dinner with my female coworkers was the cause of my feelings of embarrassment.

Why did I ditch them?

I admitted to myself that I didn't want the feeling of not belonging that often comes when a group of women get together. Everyone starts talking about their families and children, while I am a childless widow

79

(there is no word for "I lost an unmarried partner," so I used widow) with a family history riddled with drugs, suicides, and abuse. I've politely smiled my way through those long evenings. I've always felt an uncomfortable mix of jealousy and boredom as women shared their familiar stories about family and life.

Conversely, I awkwardly dealt with questions about myself because it still wasn't polite to say, "My family tried to suck the life out of me, and I was most happy when I stopped talking to my father and my mother died." I could only imagine the empty stares and awkward silences that comment would garner.

As I ate my fantastic shrimp dish and sipped some lovely wine, I realized that the feeling of unworthiness wasn't about shopping at all. It was about my living a different kind of life than my coworkers. I felt this unworthiness in me that I hadn't been *allowed* to have a life with children and extended family.

●●●●●●●●

From those kinds of memories, I learned that integration doesn't always lead to perspective shifts. Sometimes it uncovers more profound trauma points. I was aware, more than ever before, that I had these deep feelings of isolation, not belonging anywhere, and not feeling worthy of kind and caring people in my life. It would take months for me to address these feelings because they were so powerfully cruel that they ultimately motivated me to move forward with more psychedelic-assisted psychotherapy.

I didn't know that all the clues lay buried in my memories. I was too close to them. I couldn't distinguish my reality based on my early childhood experiences from how an adult would see and experience those events. I didn't make any connections.

Thankfully, my guides saw those connections like they were highlighted words on a page.

Chapter 18

Body Shame

A topic in October that swirled in my journals was my ever-present body image shame. By the third week of integration, that uncomfortable shame was front and center in my journals.

It started with a general feeling of shame for having a figure. I've always been conscious of my appearance since I was rather busty by eleven. Even though I tried to cover myself up with extra-large shirts, they were about as useful as a screen door on a submarine. Once I hit puberty, I never felt comfortable in my skin.

I had this general sense of unease and noticed I was choosing super slouchy clothes even though I was working from home and was only a head on a screen. I felt a need to cover up, so I wondered about my sense of body shame during one of Sadie's walks in the crisp fall air. My mind responded quickly with a timeline of memories that started with a feeling of shame that came along with puberty and flowed through a powerful fear of men.

●●●●●●●

I first remembered going to cheerleading practice when I was dressed in a tank top and shorts, like all the other girls. My mother looked at me and said rather acidly, "Are you going to wear that?" This seemed such a small conversation. I mean a bubble on a wave of

ocean currents, but boy, I felt a surge of shame and embarrassment come over me as Sadie and I walked down the hill. I could still see my mother's disapproving face while my stomach contracted from embarrassment. I felt like I was fourteen again.

●●●●●●●

Another time, my mother described my body to another woman as a "brick shit house." I didn't know what that meant at the time, but my mother sneered when she said it. I remember my flushed face, and if the floor could have opened and swallowed me whole, I would have willingly disappeared. All I knew from my mother's body language and voice was that she didn't like my body.

Then my memory went further back to when I was twelve. An adult male neighbor asked my mother if he could have sex with me. She, of course, said no. She told me to cover up and always have my key out so I could get into our apartment as fast as possible. We didn't know if the neighbor would take no for an answer, and my mother had no proof of the request so she didn't call the police. I learned how important it was to cover up and stay safe. Being safe was my responsibility.

●●●●●●●

Suddenly the timeline shifted to a few years later, and I confused Sadie when I stopped in my tracks and remembered how I used to find my father in my bed. I remembered he consistently over-shared about sex with his girlfriends. I grimaced with disgust when I remembered his comments about my "jiggly breasts and fat thighs" while I lived with him in my late teens.

I remembered my baggy sweats and my lack of effort with hair and make-up when I lived with him. Maybe my attire wasn't teenage depression as much as trying to keep myself as invisible as possible?

●●●●●●●

Then my memories jumped to when I was in college and three very handsy guys cornered me in a bar. I managed to get away and walked back to the dorm alone, trying to hold back my tears. I was so disappointed when I realized that danger was everywhere. Danger didn't stop when I was away from my parents. The walk back to the dorm was one of the heaviest I had ever felt. Those jerky college guys were more proof that I couldn't be comfortable just being me, and I had to camouflage myself to stay under the radar. I figured that I had to always be on guard, and hyper-aware of others

84

to protect myself.

• • • • • • •

Then, twenty-five years later, I found myself hiding in my own house to avoid my often drunk, creepy neighbor. Our condos were attached, and our front doors faced each other. He smoked and drank while he sat on his porch, so I saw him often the summer that Carl passed. There were quite a few lewd comments about how I looked and dressed. He drunkenly hit on me a few times when Sadie and I got home from our walks. In the pit of my stomach, I knew that men could be dangerous and drunk men even more so.

• • • • • • •

With these memories lumped together, I realized that I used baggy clothing to please my mother and avoid what I perceived to be dangerous male attention.

I never linked those memories together before. Now I looked at them and thought about them from my adult perspective. The body image shit from my mother was easy to shift in my head. I mean, she had shot herself, so her body image must have been low with a massive crater-like scar across her midsection. Plus, the last thing she wanted was a pregnant daughter. I understood that any issues she may have had about my body were her issues.

The fear, on the other hand, was harder to shift. My childhood had taught me that men turn abusive quickly and without warning. I was embarrassed to admit I feared my usually drunk, scowling, divorced male neighbor. Without Carl around, I didn't feel safe in my house. I was ridiculously careful to keep my doors locked all the time.

But I noticed that I saw progress when I was in public and felt safe with other women around. I won't say it was a snap of the finger, but I noticed a few weeks after that first MDMA journey, I started dressing differently for the gym. I was wearing a basic tank top and was completely ok without my baggy t-shirt. In mid-spin class, I suddenly realized I was in the front row, sweating like a maniac doing some hills, and I didn't feel a need to hide even though there were some men in the class.

Being in the front row was a small integration step, but it was a solid step towards being more comfortable being me. My tank top with, "I don't cuss, these are my workout words" was the very first hint I was changing my perspective and starting to feel more comfortable in my own skin.

Chapter 19

Sadie's New Path

One of the reasons for writing this book versus just publishing my journals is that my journals are unreadable. I mean, really unreadable. I am not exaggerating when I say I repeated ideas and questions on average five to ten times per topic. For traumatic events, I probably wrote about them more than thirty times throughout my treatment. Most of the chapters in this book were born from the perspective shifts that I saw grow through several journal entries. I didn't include the small perspective shifts or things mentioned in my journals only once or twice because, frankly, they weren't that interesting to anyone but me. Ironically, I questioned my repetition a lot in my journals. Because of my insecurity, I assumed my brain needed the extra overtime to heal. But one day, during a Sadie walk, of course, I realized the repetition wasn't a deficiency in my healing; it was the *way* to heal.

I was thinking of a way to explain how the repetition helped me change my perspective and finally looked right in front of me— at Sadie's wagging tail as she headed down the hill!

For years, Sadie's primary dog-walking path was "out the door, go to the end of the road, turn right, turn left, go around the complex, and then back home up the hill." I was on autopilot for most of those walks.

Then one beautiful sunny day, we walked out of the house, and Sadie made an immediate right. She headed to a grassy hill by the side of my row of homes. I didn't think

87

too much of it.

But I noticed that Sadie liked to walk that way because she headed in that new direction more often than not. From her perspective, I realized it made complete sense. Before, most of our walks were on concrete or asphalt. This new path was mainly grass. It must have felt much better for her aging legs, and I know I enjoyed seeing pretty trees sooner. The more Sadie trotted to the right to start our walks, the more that path became our standard path. Now I rarely even think to walk the old way. The grass-covered path makes so much more sense that it is now our regular way we do our doggie walkies.

I don't remember the draw of the old way we walked. It had just become a habit until Sadie decided to shake things up.

This repetitive shift in thinking, explained through dog walks, is precisely how my integration worked with my memories and beliefs.

The MDMA seemed to disrupt my thinking during the journey—just like how Sadie disrupted our walking path. Then during my integration, I could experience my memories from my adult perspective without my body's alarm bells going off. With enough repetition in my journals, I permanently changed my perspective about how I thought about a childhood memory (usually placing blame where it belonged) a bit more. In the same way the new dog-walking path made sense, I saw my perspective shifts as things that just made sense. In fact, without my journals to document my incremental shifts, I would have trouble remembering how I used to experience life through all my trauma lenses.

In marketing, it is commonly known that it takes seven "touches" to motivate people to some sort of action. That is another way of saying that adults need repetition to learn and absorb new information. It made sense that unraveling trauma took even more repetition for me to think differently about my fear-filled past. It took me months to stop criticizing myself for the repetition. I've included some repetition around the most significant trauma points that spanned multiple journeys to normalize how much psychedelic-assisted psychotherapy I needed to dislodge deep trauma. The more I washed and rinsed those memories in my journals, and addressed them in other journeys, the more I could make sense of them from an adult, non-trauma-influenced perspective.

Chapter 20

Going Platinum

During the end of the fourth week of my integration, the October chill forced me to live in warm sweatshirts and curl up next to my fireplace at night. My journals, however, went back to a summer, pre-journey memory.

● ● ● ● ● ● ●

My widow's fog let my father back into my life at forty-six. I don't remember how it happened, but I simply didn't care about anything after Carl's passing. So, weirdly, it didn't matter that my father was another person in my life. I knew he would have an angle, and it didn't matter. I know it seems odd considering how I spent so many years of my life afraid of him. I can't explain my thinking other than grief chips away at optimism and hope. I felt like the universe would keep using me as a punching bag. I didn't think I had much to live for at the time, and my father being my asshole father didn't matter.

And I can admit, there was a sense of keeping my enemies close. I knew my father sniffing around my life meant he wanted something. Part of me wanted to be proactive to try and see how he would try to manipulate me. I had enough of my wits about me that I could look at his behavior from afar. I wanted to know what he thought he could get from me so I wouldn't be caught off guard. I was careful and put a big, strong, high wall between us. I was the small-talk queen while listening to his hour-long barrages about his health, the terrible nurses, and doctors who "wouldn't" help him. He never figured out that I muted him for several minutes during his rants about his doctors because he wasn't interested in talking with me; he simply wanted to talk *at* me.

Soon he started sending occasional snail-mail checks. I enjoyed seeing his pattern unfold again and got a kick that he thought money had power over me like it did when I was sixteen. He had no idea how to deal with me as an adult, so he stayed on brand. I cashed those checks as soon as I got them and bought beautiful things for the house. I enjoyed the irony of his money being used to make my home, which *I* had paid for, prettier. Fancy curtains I would never buy—done!

As we headed into the summer months before my first journey, I won a fantastic award (I mean "Go to Hawaii" type of fabulous award!) at work because of my trauma-induced hypervigilant productivity. I remembered how I tapered my excitement because I didn't want the universe to find out and send something equally bad my way. After all, I learned about the prize the day before the third anniversary of Carl's death. I assumed the universe's timing was nothing short of ironic. It wanted to make sure I didn't get too big for my britches.

After the announcement, I headed to Las Vegas for a work conference, and because of the award, I got to stay at the Ritz instead of the hotel where the rest of my team stayed. Let me tell you, my twenty-year K-12 education career never prepared me for staying at a Ritz Carlton. One night I decided to go full out "bougie" and relax in the Olympic-sized tub—because—I could!

And then, my father called.

I paused for a moment before I picked up the phone. On the one hand, I was enjoying tremendous success in a life I had built without him in it. I could have easily never told him about the award. On the other hand, I was super curious about how he would react. If there was ever a time for a slam dunk "How to be a Good Parent" opportunity, this was it. All he had to do was simply congratulate me to get his three-pointer! Something inside me wanted to test him and see his reaction. Since all I talked about with him was work, it was natural to talk, with very few specifics, about the award and prizes.

Then with lovely lavender bubbles around

me and a towel pillow cradling my head, I
waited for his response. Again, he stayed on
brand.

"Can you hock any of the prizes?"

No, "Great job!" or "I'm proud of you!"
Nothing. Emptiness. I remember I
acknowledged that his reaction was his failure.
Instead, he threw another baited hook for me
to give information about my economics. If I
needed to "hock" the prizes, he would know
his regular strategy of throwing money around
might work to let me trust him again. I just
looked at that baited hook, ignored it, and let
him drone on about whatever.

●●●●●●●

I journaled about how disappointed I was in my silence. I
judged myself harshly. Here I was, an award winner in a
big tech company, and I didn't express my disappointment
in his inability to congratulate me. Instead, I let his
comments sit and let him babble. Even at the highest point
in my career, I still didn't own who I was, and I let him be
an asshole and attempt to spread his negative energy.
Thank goodness bubbles in my Olympic-sized tub stopped
his shithead energy from ruining any of my fun at the
week's award festivities.

In my October journal entries, I kept writing and
punishing myself for not speaking up during that summer
call. Remember—the interaction happened a few months
before my first journey, so of course I didn't confront him
and tell him how I felt about his comments. But after the

journey, I questioned the cost of my co-dependency on my mental health. Was I going to continue and have that shitty energy in my life because I could handle it? Or was it time to put the *CLOSED* sign on that relationship for the last time?

Interestingly, I played his "Can you hock any of the prizes?" comment in various journal entries over ten times! That is where the magic of perspective shifts became clear. Because of the repetition in my journals, I saw my progress from thinking of him as just an asshole to:

> *He must not have experienced recognition when he did good things. I assume at some point he must have done something well.*

> *I feel sorry for him; he never experienced the joy of being happy for someone else.*

> *What a shame he can't take joy in having a bright, loving, and successful daughter.*

On the surface, looking at a person or situation from a different perspective sounds so easy. I did that all the time with work challenges or financial planning, but when it came to my trauma from childhood abuse, my trapped fears were so deeply ingrained that my body never listened when any of my friends told me how much my father missed out not knowing me as an adult. Before the widow's fog, I had only felt fear, anger, and disgust when I thought about him. Without MDMA-assisted psychotherapy and my integration, I never would have felt one ounce of empathy for him. I would never have stopped looking at him from my childhood perspective.

I had always thought about keeping a physical distance from him for obvious reasons. If he wasn't around me, he couldn't hit me. But not having him in my life to protect my mental health? I never thought that way before. The MDMA therapy allowed me to be more compassionate towards myself. Maybe I deserved not to have that energy in my life versus keeping him at a distance because of my fear? Suddenly, I remembered how I protected myself from physical harm in my thirties.

●●●●●●●●

In 2010 my father discovered the Internet and learned that I worked in a school district. He called me at work. When I picked up my office extension and heard his voice, my body felt like I needed to run for my life.

I wasted no time getting some protection. I told my immediate coworkers a bit of my abuse-tinged history. I made it clear that anyone who described himself as my father should not be allowed past the lobby. I gave them enough information to clarify that it would be a genuine call for help if I called them from the parking lot. I even went so far as to give our district police liaison a description of my father, so she knew that if I called her, there was a high probability he was in the district and I was in danger.

●●●●●●●●

That memory made me realize that in my late forties, I wasn't living with that severe fear of him that I had in my early thirties. My fears had been dampened since he told me repeatedly about his health issues. He couldn't come after me with hard fists the way he had when he was younger. He couldn't suddenly appear in a parking lot and attack me. Maybe it was now time to put me first and protect my mental health with the energy I used to protect my physical safety for all those years?

It turned out that empathy towards myself was the superpower to release some of my trapped emotions. Yes, he was an asshole, and I didn't forget his abuse. But being able to distance myself from those childhood feelings and memories let me see him from afar as if he were a friend's father. That perspective clarified my father's behavior in a way that I never saw before.

I even wrote at one point:

Hey, is it worth being scared of the pathetic?

Chapter 21

Jazz Hand Slaps

I rarely heard the inner voice around mid-October, unless I was super relaxed and tried to create a conversation. I would get quiet and say, "Hi" while I walked Sadie. Sometimes my Type A personality would chill out and let a conversation happen, but I was too focused on work to make any progress most of the time. The act of looking inward was a challenging new behavior for me.

So one blustery afternoon during a regular dog walk, I wanted to see if I could start a conversation and hesitantly asked, "Hi?"

I didn't hear a voice, but my mind shifted quickly to wonder why I lived with so many people after my mother shot herself.

●●●●●●●

I remembered how my mother was in no condition to care for me when I was young. She was recovering from her shotgun wound, going to lots of doctors, and trying to get her feet under her. She self-medicated along with her prescriptions to try and dislodge her numbing depression. When I visited her, I knew that there wasn't room for me in her life.

For whatever reason, I also didn't live with my father during those years. Did he not have an apartment? Did he not have a job? Did he

97

not want to be a single dad? I never asked him why I lived with relatives all that time. It suddenly occurred to me that he clearly didn't have his shit together either. Since he never talked about those years when I only saw him occasionally, I never knew his story.

●●●●●●●

It was hard to cobble together, but I think I lived in three homes from ages five to eight. I have vague memories of being with extended family, but I couldn't remember for how long and at what ages.

As Sadie and I got to the bottom of the hill, I realized that my transient early years were probably because my father was a lot to take. Why the heck didn't I stay with one family? Why didn't my father let his sister care for me since she had two children and had offered (I learned later) to take me?

I'm guessing that aside from any financial burden of feeding me, he acted like no one could do anything right, and that probably got old with my relatives. He could rival anyone on any cheapskates television show with his own dumpster diving. And, of course, his "all about me 24/7" personality probably annoyed everyone. There was a ton of extended family on my father's side that I never knew because my father was just so miserable; nobody kept in touch with him.

Before this little inner conversation, I had just taken it for granted that the universe wouldn't let me stay settled. Something about *me* and my lack of worth caused the constant upheaval. I didn't know at that young age that my father could barely keep a job, and my mother was healing a gaping wound in her stomach while dealing with drugs and depression issues. I just knew what I knew from a child-centric view:

I wasn't *good enough* to stay in one place.

I didn't deserve a family.

I didn't deserve friends.

I didn't deserve to be happy.

Other kids got those things.

While Sadie sniffed around, I realized how much I was shuffled around had little to do with me and everything to do with my parents. They didn't have their shit together. I smiled as that realization came to me as manicured, jazz-hand-mini-forehead-slap. Of course, they didn't have their shit together! I never had a conversation about that time in my life to rethink it before. Now, from my adult perspective, it was stunningly clear that I wasn't the reason I got shuffled around. I certainly didn't bring any of that on myself, and my feelings of worthlessness were wholly misplaced.

But I still felt physically uncomfortable thinking about my worth. It was like my body just didn't feel right.

I wish that jazz-hand-mini-forehead-slap had been an emotional lightning bolt. This perspective shift around my transient years helped me understand why I felt so pessimistic about the future but shifting this perspective didn't take those nasty feelings away.

While I was enjoying these shifts, sometimes it felt overwhelming, and I doubted I could fully heal some of these deeply embedded thoughts. Plus, in the back of my mind, I was just a little bit scared. After all, my thoughts about myself had been part of me for so long, who would I be without them?

Chapter 22

Big Britches

I had been searching for a new house for over a year. I felt a constant mental zigzag between wanting to stay and needing to move. On the one hand, I had my comfortable little condo with so many beautiful memories of Carl. On the other hand, I was getting increasingly ready to close that chapter of my life and start fresh in a new house.

One night, while Zillow surfing through house listings, I heard:

> **Inner Voice:** You don't deserve it.

I questioned this voice since it wasn't very nice. Why didn't I deserve a house? I had been in a comfortable suburban home for twenty years, and I never felt like I didn't deserve to be here. Then I heard:

> **Male Inner Voice:** You'll get too big for your britches.

This wasn't my father; he never used that language. I don't know where I had heard it. As I tried to figure out the origin of that line in my history, suddenly I heard a snide comment from the same voice.

> **Male Inner Voice:** Who do you think you are?

That question flowed through me like a dunk in a cold

ocean and left me feeling ashamed. I didn't know what I was ashamed of, but I knew how my body felt. And oddly, I could not figure out who that voice was or the first time I heard it. I can't even be sure those words were ever spoken to me or if I internalized my father's hateful vocabulary as *truth*.

I pulled my sofa blankie closer around me and cuddled with Sadie. But that wasn't enough to loosen my tight shoulders or ease my stomach that had just flipped.

I didn't have anything to counteract those thoughts. It was like they were weights strapped to my ankles, and they pulled me down into freezing water. My whole body felt heavy. I was stuck with the feelings left from hearing that male voice. I had over twenty-five years of life experience to disprove those feelings, but that voice was there—stuck in my head. That was how my PTSD kept me captive.

This feeling of shame came over me, just like my feelings of isolation. I wasn't expecting either one of those feelings to be so strong. They grabbed my focus. The feelings were suddenly right in front of my awareness. Everything else in my life, like work and Sadie, was tinged with those emotions. I felt like the MDMA journey had allowed these emotions to climb into my consciousness while I had always managed to keep them pushed down with hyperactivity and overthinking to survive life.

That night I emailed my guides and asked for a second journey. I summarized all the integration work I had done and the emotions that I couldn't control. I pointed out that I had been able to identify my negative thought patterns instead of blindly believing them. I asked my therapist if we could focus on these feelings during our talk therapy sessions. I hoped I could craft some intentions around them.

I even joked with my guides that I wouldn't lock them out of my mental house as I did on the first journey. I told them the doors would be unlocked, and I would offer them unlimited drinks and hors d'oeuvres if they would help me with a second journey. While my therapist promised me that we could do more work if my one journey didn't heal all my trauma, I totally forgot all of that and felt like I had to convince them to work with me. My therapeutic journeys were a full day of work for everyone involved. To me, a full eight hours of working with me was a very serious ask.

I crossed my fingers that we could find a time in December. I found myself impatient because, for the first time, I understood psychedelic-assisted psychotherapy could provide me relief. I didn't know what it would take, but I knew I didn't want to live the rest of my life with these intense feelings of isolation and shame as my primary emotions.

I didn't know that the same way they simply guided me while I was medicated was also their way to help me with my integrations. They waited for me to ask for a second journey because only I would know when I was ready for another dose and more integration work. I didn't realize it at the time, but I had worked within their unspoken parameters that let me direct my healing timeline.

All I knew was relief that we managed to coordinate our calendars for the end of December.

Chapter 23

Cabinets in Peril

By the end of October, I rarely chatted with my inner voice. Maybe two times a week I would hear a comment or two, but I wasn't having insightful conversations like at the beginning of my integration. I had made lots of progress, but old routines and survival strategies came back like riding a bike. As usual, I spent the bulk of my time working. In my job, every day was different, and I enjoyed solving problems. I don't like migraine-level projects all the time but didn't mind having my head occasionally hurt with figuring out solutions that made sense for partners and customers. Plus, working equaled continued survival for me, so it was my natural pattern, and I considered myself lucky that I enjoyed my career.

My journals showed my growth as I integrated my journey into my daily life. I could choose how I felt about the little things in life as they happened because I saw those little things differently than I ever had before. It was like when I watched the movie *Shrek* for the second time, and I saw more of the bawdy humor. It was the same movie, with the same storyline, but I almost spit out my drink the second time around when I saw the naked cartoon king checking himself out under his sheet.

That is precisely how some of my childhood memories played out during this time. I was able to see different details about them than I saw as a child. Without my body responding to my fears I had when I was a child, I could concentrate a lot more on the specifics I had never thought about before.

Usually, my memory replays were relatively mild. I was repetitively writing about my memories and exploring different viewpoints with my computer on my lap and hot tea close by.

But occasionally this process was unexpected and explosive. When the second-longest relationship of my life was on the verge of ending, I had an over-the-top emotional reaction.

My boyfriend and I were control freaks who couldn't seem to meet in the middle. I had met him about two months after my hospital stay when I decided to get my shit together. I never expected an actual relationship to happen that quickly, but a bright, kind, handsome man, who also worked in technology, walked into my life. He knew where I was emotionally; I learned where he was emotionally, and then suddenly, we were a couple for a few years.

I've always believed in the idea of soul mates not only being couples. They can be mentors, teachers, doctors, and even trusted neighbors. I've learned that there are some people with whom I feel a strong connection. So, while I knew in my heart that this man and I were soul mates, that didn't mean that we could couple for the rest of our lives.

And I was sad. Sadness was the expected emotion. But the next day after our talk, the unexpected feeling that surged across my shoulders was anger. I was steaming fucking angry! I mean, loud temper tantrums in the checkout lane because I didn't get my candy, angry. My internal voice showed up while I tried to figure out these emotions because I had stomped around my kitchen and slammed every cabinet. The innocent microwave was next.

This breakup was a joint decision we were making. Why

was I so angry?

This man hadn't taken advantage of me, hadn't cheated on me, and hadn't done anything wrong.

So why the anger? Why the cacophony of cabinet slams?

While standing in front of the microwave waiting for my tea water to heat up (Oh, stop judging. I was in no mood to wait for my kettle), I called to my inner voice:

> **Jill:** Can't I be happy once he leaves?
> **Inner Voice:** I'm going to be alone.
> **Jill:** What does that mean? He and I don't live together. Since COVID, I have spent most of my time alone.
> **Inner Voice:** I'm going to have to work doubly hard.
> **Jill:** Why?
> **Inner Voice:** To stay hidden, so nothing bad happens.

As my tea steeped, I felt a full-body flush of fear, and I remembered how scary life was when I was nineteen and... *alone.*

At this point, I realized I was integrating my past with my present because I remembered when I was nineteen with one year of college behind me.

● ● ● ● ● ● ●

A month after I turned nineteen, I was home from my first year of college. My father thought he could hit me as he had done throughout my childhood.

I remember studying in my room for a

105

horrendous geology summer course to get some core credits out of the way. My father came into the room, and while I don't remember what we argued about—I remembered how he leaned over and slapped me across the face. My memories are a weird mix of a textbook page of rocks and the sting of his slap on my cheek.

A year away from him made that first and last slap sting hard because I had let my guard down. A year away at college had let me focus on the usual first-year student's fears around grades and finances. I didn't expect to get slapped at all that summer, let alone the first week I was home. I was a college student, for fuck's sake, and with all the pride I held in that title, something in me snapped.

I remembered his surprised face when I stood up with my flaming red cheek. I made eye contact without crying. I didn't attack him or insult him. I stared at him and somehow communicated that I would not get hit again. He left the room with a door slam.

I wasn't relieved he left, though. I was terrified, and my whole body shook as my adrenaline surged. I knew he would simmer at my bravery and come back even angrier. That slap was a test—to see how much control he still had. I knew he was going to come back stronger and more furious. When my mother tried to stand up for herself before she shot herself, my father punched her so many times that he shattered her eardrum.

Luckily, he left the apartment quickly. I called my mother and begged her to let me stay with her until I could get myself settled. At the time, I knew I was trading a college education for my safety.

It was a no-brainer.

I left his apartment with one hastily packed suitcase and went to my mother's apartment. This time, when he came around, she hid me. In super stalker style, he would show up at all hours, banging on the door looking for me on random days. My mother and I had learned our lesson. He wasn't going to take anything from either one of us ever again.

As life moved on, my mother remarried and moved to another state. I was on my own. I was in a crappy apartment and worked two shitty jobs, but I was on my own, not getting hit or verbally abused.

I still felt trapped and incredibly vulnerable, though. My father was famous for just showing up. During those eighteen months I lived with him, he was rarely employed, so he would drop in during my after-school activities. He would drop in at work and routinely verify my schedule. Like domestic abusers, he tried to give me the illusion that he always knew where I was. It made sense that I lived a bit paranoid at nineteen. I knew he

could show up unexpectantly and that if he did, I wasn't physically strong enough to fight him off.

●●●●●●●

Those years when I was nineteen to twenty-four were when I felt weak and scared. Even though I eventually got myself back to college by working two jobs and living on pasta, I was terrified during those years of losing everything. I knew my father could find me and hurt me. No matter how strong I appeared on the surface by being on my own and working like a maniac to get my college degree, inside I was a terrified toddler who very slowly grew up. It took years of small academic successes and relationships without abuse to feel a bit safer in the world.

I didn't want that fucking life! I didn't want to go through that again! Being alone and having to do everything! Being scared and constantly looking over my shoulder! I didn't want the stress of living like my life was on the line every single minute of the day. I was spitting angry about it!

I stepped back from the microwave dumbfounded that I made this super weird assumption that my life would revert to what it was like at nineteen. Why?

> **Inner Voice:** I will be all alone again.
> **Jill:** Really?

Silence...
Suddenly my shoulders relaxed, and I took a deep breath. My mind showed me I was in a vastly different place than I was at nineteen. I was no longer hiding from my father. I didn't have to be angry that I didn't have a man in my life

to protect me from my father. If my father wanted to create chaos, I would deal with it.

And, most importantly, he wouldn't win.

I survived Carl's death, I was financially stable, and I had close friends who would bring the cavalry. I even knew a fellow dog parent police officer right around the corner. My handy cell phone could record at a moment's notice if my father suddenly showed up. He could finally be held accountable if he tried to hurt me.

I wasn't alone or struggling. I was no longer a domestic abuse victim who needed to be afraid of her father.

Nope, I was an adult who could fend for herself! He was old and feeble. He was not a threat. His only weapon was manipulation, which I could see from a mile away when we talked.

My thoughts were exactly what a stable, loving parent would have said while I stood in the kitchen. In essence, I did a little reparenting while getting my green tea ready. I talked to my inner nineteen-year-old and calmed her the fuck down.

And, instead of being an ornery teenager, she listened!

My raging anger disappeared. Initially started by my MDMA journey, this perception shift was a massive integration flag in the sand for my healing! I sipped my tea and moved on to the day's tasks without harming any more innocent cabinets.

Chapter 24

November's Ass-Kicking

While my journals showed my integration successes, they also revealed new layers of trauma. It became clear that I could make progress *and* see more work I had to do, often in the same journal entry.

With its shorter days and cold winds, November rolled around. While the wind howled outside and always seemed to pick up during dog walks, my internal shame about my childhood broiled white-hot inside me.

I was always embarrassed by my childhood. I had in my head that anyone coming from a background like mine was defective, and I had to hide that part of me. It had taken me years to share with Carl all my crazy background, and I didn't tell my boyfriend anything until months after we started seeing each other, and only after lots of prodding.

I think part of my hyper-productivity was my way to prove I was "normal" and that I wasn't inept at life like my parents. Being successful in my career, according to my terms, was especially important to me. I think my own purpose has always been defined by my ability to help other people and has been the common thread throughout my career choices. My hyper-productivity at work, to help others, was a way I could feel better about myself. I didn't let outside factors like school board meetings or quotas impact my behavior. I always just competed against myself with my personal metric being how much of an impact I had made to help people in some way.

But I always thought people would figure out I was

knitting my life with only one needle. I thought I was fortunate that I found Carl, who I always thought had *overlooked* my background and loved me for me. He didn't have my level of trauma, so he accepted me for the loving and kind person he saw in front of him. I just never thought of our relationship that way.

While journaling to a prompt about the importance of self-love, my mind spiraled into a shame attack about getting mental health treatment. My internal conversation was brutal.

> **Jill:** What if they (guides) figure out I'm not worth it and stop helping me?
> **Inner Voice:** Why would they do that? This is a treatment that needs a few go-arounds (journeys), and they are leaning in to help you. Why would they stop?
> **Jill:** Because I can't fool them anymore.
> **Inner Voice:** Fool them about what?
> **Jill:** How weak I am that I can't stop my mind from how I think. I'm not good enough.

In my journal, I asked myself some tough questions:

> *Am I a weak person?*
> *Is there any indication that my guides are suddenly going to drop me?*
> *Am I not good enough?*

Just like in school, when I was in "test-taking" mode, I should have gotten an A+ on my answers because I wrote great journal entries about my life where I was strong and indeed *good enough*. My guides weren't going to drop me;

they had been supportive and receptive through the entire process. And dang it, if the life I had led so far hadn't proved I was a good person at heart—well then, I had nothing left to offer.

Yet, I couldn't change my thought patterns or the deep, queasy feeling in my stomach even with my detailing work success after work success. Even with multiple journal entries, I felt weak and unworthy of this treatment. These were my regular thinking patterns that felt like cold, wet, heavy mud-soaked blankets. Those patterns always pulled me backward; they stopped me from moving forward, and I had no idea what life would be like without them because I used them to protect me from getting hurt my whole life. It was easier to feel the shame of doubting myself first and staying small rather than risking shining and the universe slapping back at me to *keep me in my place*.

No one was going to hurt me worse than I hurt myself.

My guides warned me that my unresolved trauma would probably make me emotional before my second journey in December. The ways my mind protected me as a child would be brutal to dislodge, and they told me to expect "lots of things to come up." The therapy avoidance strategy of "I am just so bad no one would want to work with me" was an interesting mind fuck, though. That was the strategy my scared inner children used to avoid anyone messing with their mental apple carts.

The self-descriptive word *defective* showed up way too many times in those November journals. I didn't know where that feeling came from, but I knew it didn't feel good. I cried almost every time I journaled because those terrible feelings of just not being good enough for anything were constantly in my head and heart.

I was beyond frustrated that I couldn't figure out *why* I

felt defective.

I journaled and cried my way through November while I did my best in my bi-weekly talk therapy sessions to craft my next journey's intentions.

Chapter 25

Bring on the Binge

In late November 2020, I spoke to my father for the last
time. At the time of this writing, we haven't talked since.

During that last call, my father told me that he had eaten
Thanksgiving dinner at the VA and went to "a lot of
trouble" to tell the newer vets how to navigate the system.
He spent "so much time" explaining the processes, and
these guys "couldn't get enough of it," so he'll be making
the "two-hour drive" to "help out those guys" next week.
As always, I listened, being thankful that I hadn't spent
Thanksgiving with him. I hadn't shared any holiday with
my father during my adulthood.

Then boom! Fifteen minutes after getting off the phone
with him, I gorged on sugar-laden, processed crap. I threw
open the cabinets and found *all* the "treat food" that makes
my blood sugar skyrocket. I ate so many cookies and
packages of apple pies that my stomach recoiled, and I
threw up hard. This was legit worm-at-the-bottom-of-a-
tequila-bottle barf level. My stomach couldn't handle the
handfuls of junk I ate because of that conversation I had
with my father.

My jealousy of him trying to help other people was
palatable. After all the pain and abuse he threw at my
mother and me, I felt his stories of being helpful to others
as insults. And yet, while I could understand he was fucked
up, I chowed down enough shitty food to make *me* sick. I
needed to be full and comforted. I turned to sugar for the
dopamine and lots of it. Somewhere inside me was a

childhood Jill hurting for her father's affection.

What happened? This was an absolute PTSD reaction. I knew it while it was happening. I just couldn't stop eating.

That feeling of not being loved, or even tolerated, by this parent made me desperate to feel full, warm, and safe. The irony? His help was usually terrible, and he always wanted something in return. As an adult, I had no interest in any help from him. But somewhere inside me, I was jealous and hurt that he talked about helping others.

I was ashamed of my emotional reaction. While I lived my life inwardly responding to an undercurrent of fear this man had created, after this phone call, I reacted emotionally to him by harming my own body. It was proof of me *still* not getting over the pain he caused me, and I was ashamed. I even had trouble telling my therapist and guide about it.

My journal entry about this call and junk food binge ended with a clear intention for the second journey. My guides encouraged me to investigate my relationship with food. It was that simple. Why did I turn to sugar when I was upset? What was that sugar high giving me? When I actively tried to reduce how many processed foods I ate, what emotion was so strong to override all my frontal lobe's health goals?

Intention: What is my relationship with food?

Of course, I knew there was a more significant issue than the food. That was my body's symptom that something else was wrong. But I wanted to figure out this food issue so I didn't have to hire a personal assistant to follow me around and knock chocolate chip cookies out of my hands for the rest of my life.

Chapter 26

Second Journey Preparation

My 40% talk therapy portion for the second journey consisted of sessions with my therapist in November and December and at least one session with my therapist and guide. We never started those sessions with any "let's talk about your childhood" prompts. Instead, we focused on what major or minor struggles I brought to the conversations. Silly things that upset me in my day-to-day life were quickly peeled back and revealed beliefs crafted from the years of childhood abuse and neglect. I was the most surprised when minor work frustrations pointed to foundational trauma issues. I remember finally understanding one of my therapist's favorite statements, "As adults, we are all little children wrapped in layers." Probably, for the first time, I realized that my unresolved childhood hurts directed many of my adult thoughts and feelings.

Those sessions were some of the best talk therapy hours I have ever had. Most importantly, I learned that if I felt embarrassed about something, that was just the tip of a trauma iceberg. There was a whole lot of trouble under the surface that I couldn't see. I was so caught up in my weird shame loops, and it took a lot of work for me to "own up" to embarrassing or shameful thoughts. My guides always took those conversations in stride, and I realized that while I thought my shame-filled thoughts were rated R, my guides had the correct perspective and gave those feelings the appropriate G rating. During our therapy chats, my guides practically rubbed their hands together in glee because they knew the more shame I brought to our conversations, the more I could heal.

I admit to a bit of shame in one of our pre-journey talk therapy sessions:

————

Jill: I have these intentions, and I am embarrassed to work on them because I feel like I am cheating.
Therapist: Cheating?
Jill: Well, I have done some work, and I feel like I understand what is causing some of those behaviors, so I should slog through and keep figuring things out. I'm cheating by going for a second experience to give me more clarity. At some point, the universe will smack my hand for wanting too much.
Therapist: Why aren't you allowed to get more help? Why aren't you allowed to try and heal these hurts?
Jill: Because that isn't how the universe works. I slog through despite the universe. (Pause) But that hasn't been the case for the last twenty-five years. I'm not sure why I still feel this way.

————

At this point, just like during the first journey's integration, my mind used memories to explain the origin of my thoughts and feelings. Our conversation shifted to my mother, and I thought about her sad life choices. I realized I had this weird assumption that my life followed the same miserable path my mother's life had taken. My mother lived with her parents and then with her abusive husband. After their divorce, she battled with mental illness, drugs, and poverty for the rest of her life. Her second marriage ended in a medical bankruptcy that everyone warned her would happen. She always managed to make decisions that prevented joy.

But, so far, my life didn't follow her format of failure and neediness. I always thought the idea that the universe would keep me in check and not let me get too happy was from my father's abuse. It turns out; I also internalized my mother's unhappy life as the prime example that I couldn't live any better. I don't think my mother ever knew that she had a choice to be happy.

Looking at my mother's life differently was just one example of how vital the pre-journey talk therapy sessions were. Sometimes I had amazing breakthroughs, like the realization about my mother's life. Other times I openly tackled a deeply shameful issue that left me feeling queasy and anxious as the issue floated around my thoughts for days before the journey. I was deeply embarrassed to keep asking for help. I was deeply embarrassed that two brilliant people were putting effort into helping me, and I wasn't knocking my healing out of the park. Plus, I doubted the universe would even let me keep healing.

Yet all I got from my guides were smiles, encouraging words, and even homework for our subsequent sessions. They were in if I was in!

Chapter 27

Setting Intentions

Before the second journey, I felt like a mental storm was brewing in my head and body. Before the first MDMA journey, I was nervous and scared because my Type A-ness focused on my ability to do the journey *correctly*. Getting ready for the second MDMA journey, however, was more challenging. In early December, the two weeks before the journey, I had massive amounts of brain fog and had tears in my eyes more often than not. I had a general feeling of cold gloom like I couldn't take off a soaked, icicle-laced parka.

Two weeks before the journey, my guides gave me homework to flesh out my intentions in our last talk therapy session. They used content from our chats and turned them into questions. For instance, the first homework assignment was to notice and detail when I felt unworthy. I needed to remember what was happening in my life if I flushed with embarrassment for no reason. I needed to document when I thought, "Oh, I couldn't possibly do X, Y, and Z," because it would put me in the spotlight, and I'm not worth it. Since I didn't feel worthy of even getting my guides' help, these were excellent assignments to see how often those thoughts swirled in my head.

I wrote acres of digital journals about my career growth and impostor syndrome in completing my assignments. All the preparation, the grit, and hard work that got me to where I am in life made it clear that I had no reason to be

119

shy about my success. With hard work and lots of hours, I had earned the right to be precisely where I was! All those Internet hustle memes about focusing and working toward goals were true in my case and allowed me to jump at career opportunities. It was a lovely, jazz-handed forehead slap of evidence right in front of me. I just needed help getting my subconscious to believe I had earned my success.

Intention: Stop feeling I'm not good enough.

The second homework assignment was, "Are you putting all the power of how you think about yourself in other people?" That was a tough one to admit I had done most of my life, and that was the advantage of having my guides walk me through these feelings. Without their gentle pushes, I would *never* have approached this homework assignment. The first time I tackled it, I had to stop and take a social media binge to disassociate and relieve my tight shoulders. I knew I always looked to others to tell me, "How am I doing?" instead of listening to my gut to tell me I was okay.

It was clear through my journaling that I didn't trust my judgment very often. I often referred to my world-shattering experience at sixteen. Letting my father back in my life shaped how I felt about my decision-making abilities. I was clearly shitty, very shitty at making decisions. If I made bad decisions, then it made sense why I depended on other people's opinions of me to signpost how I was doing. After all, my own opinion, which could lead to a decision, couldn't be trusted. The last twenty-five years of excellent decision-making, academic achievements, and career success didn't exist in those journals. It was almost like those years didn't happen, and my mind did some sort of weird time warp to skip over them. I still had those trapped emotions from when I was sixteen, and my body only paid attention to those emotions.

This lack of faith in myself was a significant factor in my fear of the future. Since I depended so much on other people to validate how I thought about myself, it made sense I couldn't muster any bravery in facing an unknown future. Other people could tell me things would work out which made things better. Carl calmed my fears for years. But at the end of the day, since I didn't trust myself, I didn't trust that I *could* make a promising future for myself.

Intention: Get rid of my fear of the future.

The last intention was pretty easy. After talking to my father, I told my guides about my sugar binge. I was so curious about why, while I had apples and bananas on the counter, that I gorged on the crappiest food I could find in the cabinets. It was like half of me watched me eat that crap, and the other half of me *needed* that crap.

Intention: What is my relationship to food?

It was good that I spent time journaling to organize my intentions because my brain was scattered the two weeks before the journey. I was super excited about the journey and couldn't wait to get back to the room with all its art and comfy blankets. I knew I would get further this time— I was sure of it! Even though many of my feelings were shame laden and hard to admit, I wanted the relief of finally putting down some heavy emotional bags in a safe, therapeutic environment.

Chapter 28

Air Bubbles

The main difference between the first and second MDMA journey was my trust in the process. I had seen the healing potential in September and looked forward to making more progress the second time around. I felt as excited as I did when I was six and eagerly climbed back onto the diving board after surviving my first terrifying dive in the pool's deep end.

I trusted my guides; they knew I had shame issues around my intentions. I knew that these two people would not inflict any pain. I remember saying, "Just be nice no matter what I say." That's where I asked permission to express every piece of bile or horrific memory that would put people off in polite conversation. They knew that what I judged to be terrible thoughts were natural responses to my childhood experiences. They could see the whole map of my trauma behavior while I was glued to the next turn on the GPS.

I was also more curious about how my mind responded to MDMA. I wanted to be "awake" for more of the journey and "see" my brain's neuroplasticity in action. I didn't have the recorded transcript of the first journey yet, and I didn't remember much of it. My inner teacher (I taught high school students early in my career) wanted to understand how this therapy influenced my brain. I'll admit, a part of me wanted to understand it so I could shortcut the process and make more progress. Type A to the Max = Jill!

Unfortunately, our journey coincided with one of the

area's worst snowstorms of the year. My therapist couldn't dig out. I was so eager to use the holiday break for processing and journaling that I asked my guide if we could brave the elements and go ahead anyway. With shovels and salt at the ready, my guide agreed!

After digging trenches to make sure we could get our cars out, we shed our snow boots and started chatting as we got settled. The journey room was as welcoming as the first time I was there. The faint smell of sage and the heater to combat the snowy day relaxed me. I was bundled up in my fleece winter layers and happily put on my thickest, comfiest socks. I felt like I had packed the perfect backpack for the first day of school. Comfy socks? Check! Eye mask? Check! Fruit, nuts, and water? Check!

My guide reminded me to relax and let the medicine do its work. The more relaxed and receptive I was to the medicine, the better the results. I was nervous that I wouldn't relax enough, and I commented about the irony of being worried about needing to relax!

We again sat in the seating area, and I explained my intentions. I liked running my intentions by my guide before the journey. Doing so felt weirdly liberating because I finally got to share my inner struggles with someone. While I was embarrassed that I had issues to resolve, here was my time to work on those issues.

This time was also an opportunity to contribute something personal to the space if I chose to. I loved this idea. I liked being able to contribute something to the healing energy of the room. In a way, even to mark that I was there, I brought some flowers from the house that wilted way too soon on my first journey. This time, I wanted to leave something more permanent and meaningful.

I had framed a Haiku written for me at a work event the same year Carl passed.

Thank the crucible
Praise the great heat that transforms
Every masterpiece

At eye level on my refrigerator, this little poem reminded me that hard things in life were teachers for the next stage of life. Those difficult teachers deserved my thanks. There was going to be life after losing Carl, and there was going to be life after confronting my childhood. The work wouldn't be easy; it would burn and hurt, but it would end, and there would be life after. Maybe my masterpiece would be a life not tinged with fear?

Then my guide steered the conversation to the concept of separation. My guide tried to explain that sometimes children take responsibility for things in their lives over which they have no control. My guide also called it a "break." I had a break wherein, with my child-centric view, I thought I could control my parents enough to not fuck up my sixteen-year-old world and future.

I wasn't buying what was being sold. Didn't he see that *I* caused my life to be upended when I was sixteen?

I fully believed it was *my* fault that I couldn't work or manipulate my parents enough for them to be nice to each other and focus on me.

I couldn't see that break because I was still stuck in the emotions of that trauma point when I was sixteen. Even with the integration after the first journey where I questioned why my father did what he did, I still felt that *I* fucked up big when I was sixteen. I couldn't bring home the gold to the Olympic Crazy Parent Games for which I had trained my whole life.

The first journey let me start seeing my parents as individuals with their own trauma. That was a significant first step, but my feelings from that day when I was sixteen were still trapped within me and directed how I thought about the world. My guides heard that loud and clear in our talk-therapy sessions.

I didn't let my minor disagreement with my guide stop me from taking the MDMA capsules. I just chalked up the conversation to another person who didn't get it. I was responsible for letting my parents fuck up my future.

Because of the cold, I quickly asked to lie down and snuggle under the covers. I found comfort in the weight of multiple blankets. Then I tried to go inward, sinking into darkness with my eye mask on, far more than I did in the first journey. But of course, surprising no one who knows me, I chatted with my guide throughout the day.

The differences between my two journeys were tremendous. With my focus on remembering more and my guide's notes, I felt more a part of the process versus the process happening to me. I remember "rambling" about topics that I didn't think related to the intentions. I even remember wondering why the MDMA had me going in these "unnecessary" directions during the journey. Even while the MDMA was doing its job, I looked at its work and wondered why it touched specific memories. Again, I didn't have any fancy visuals. The journey was one extended conversation where sometimes I chatted internally with myself and sometimes with my guide.

My guide sent his written notes to me after the journey, and it seemed like I spewed a lot of puzzle pieces that didn't quite fit together. Trying to "see" more of the journey as it happened didn't work too well for me. I got too curious about what I was chatting about and then doubted I was doing decent work. I learned that I could be more aware during journeys if I wanted to, but I wondered if doing so somehow hindered the MDMA in my system.

My trust in the process allowed me to let the journey run its full course. Remember, I cut the first journey short, which was a sign of how closed I was to the process. I thought it was an immediate win that I had relaxed enough to end the experience naturally. After about seven hours, my guide knew we were almost finished when I sat up and asked for a snack.

After spending plenty of time relaxing and noshing on fruit and nuts, we bundled up and headed to our cars. While I warmed up my car, I thanked the universe for heated seats and again doubted that work had been done. From what I remembered, the journey had seemed so scattered. I couldn't link my intentions to what I had discussed while the medicine was in my system. I'm not sure why, but I expected immediate insights and felt a little disappointed. I think it might have been a sign of how excited I was to get another shot at healing. We ended our day after we pulled out of the parking lot and gave each other the "I'm ready to drive in snow" thumbs up.

Then as I drove home, my brain brought me the image of a submerged tire. I saw tiny air bubbles floating from the tire through the water highlighting unseen pinholes. Suddenly I was a lot less judgmental about how my mind worked for the last few hours. I understood my brain's message loud and clear. My mind was the tire. The water was the MDMA which pinpointed subconscious feelings and memories that linked to my intentions. Just like tiny streams of air bubbles floating through water show pinpoint holes in tires, the MDMA had identified what I would need to work on during my integration. I just had to trust the process.

I smiled knowing that I would be dusting off and healing many old memories in the following days and weeks.

With this newfound kindness toward my healing, I drove home excited about how much I would get accomplished this time around.

Chapter 29

Integration - Journey Night

After I got home from the journey, my snow-trapped therapist checked in. I wasn't journaling at that point, but one thing from that conversation stayed with me and frustrated me for months.

My relationship to food intention got an answer immediately.

I was really excited when I told my therapist, "My weight is a made-up problem."

On the surface, my weight being a problem I created was just so obvious yet fascinating. *I* ate the crap. *I* didn't like what I looked like in specific clothing. *I* was the one who could make changes. Yet I rarely did when I was stressed. I understood that I had created this problem. There wasn't anything *wrong* with me. It wasn't about willpower. Food was a made-up problem that was related to something else entirely.

That was it. That was as far as I got on that intention, and I didn't deal with it at all in the following months of my integration work.

I mention this aborted perspective-shifting because my healing could only happen as fast as I would allow it. My psychedelic-assisted psychotherapy wasn't a magic wand. The medicine dealt with what I could deal with per journey. There was much more to my weight struggles because they spoke to an entirely different trauma issue that I didn't realize until months after my third journey. My healing went at its own pace regardless of how much I wanted my jeans to fit.

Even though I didn't resolve this trauma by the end of the third journey, that is, by the end of this book, I wanted to mention the issue to stay true to my timeline. I had a deeply embedded trauma that I couldn't identify until I healed less intense traumas. There was a pyramid of trauma in my head, and this weight issue was part of the large base. I had a lot more layers to heal before I could approach this issue.

Chapter 30

Perspective Shift – Age Sixteen

Since the food question was answered so quickly, I wasn't surprised that my first journal entry, after my second journey, was full of Pop Rock energy! While my integration was slow and steady after the first journey, my mind wasted no time cleaning up some of my shittiest beliefs about myself this second time around. While I thought I rambled my way through the journey, the MDMA had been super smart because I was raring to heal some old hurts the next day!

The day after the second journey, with hot chocolate by my side to combat the still snowy weather, I wrote a digital novel about when I was sixteen and how much that trauma influenced my life. I had lived my life with a sign around my neck warning me that I had the decision-making skills of a squirrel crossing a busy street. I was always overwhelmed and terrified by big and small decisions.

The conversation I had with my guide before the journey—about separation—was obviously on point. Before the journey, I *knew* it was *my* fault that my life was blown up when I was sixteen. One of the saddest things I said during the first journey was:

> **Jill:** Everything went away at sixteen. Scholarships went away. Personal safety went away. Boundaries went away. Faith in the future went away.

My journal now showed a major reframe. I noticed how

130

much my trauma from when I was sixteen influenced so much of my adult behavior. I reframed that trauma point to a new adult perspective in these journal segments. It was common for me to talk about my younger ages in the third person. To me, they lived in my subconscious at the ages of their trauma.

> *My inner sixteen-year-old works to protect me (anxiety, over-thinking, responding to any minor threat). She is still making up hard for her decision to trust her mother and father not to blow up her life.*
>
> *I've got to thank my inner sixteen-year-old, and she can finally stand down. She has paid me back 1000-fold. She kept me safe my entire adult life.*

The journal went on to look at my father's behavior during the eighteen months I lived with him. This might have been the first time I tried to understand my father's real motivations behind his abusive behavior. Even today, I don't know his plan when he only had a one-bedroom apartment and lacked a steady income. Something in him said, "I'm going to fuck with Jill's life" or "I am going to fuck with my ex-wife," and I honestly don't know what it was. But it was all about him. He found power by breaking people he thought were weak. I never saw him insult a man—ever.

I continued to reframe that my father's behavior had nothing to do with me as a person and instead was the result of his issues. Most importantly, I questioned the severity of his need to hurt people versus his need to break my mother and me. Asking those questions was a significant turning point as I started to Google abusive parents and narcissistic personalities for the first time. I

131

realized his wonky behavior wasn't confined to my mother and me. I don't remember him having friends, and his extended family stayed away. We just happened to be in his life and, by living with him, got the brunt of his violence and abuse.

Then, like my mind decided to turn a page, my writing shifted to people who helped me in my career. I wrote about one of my fantastic managers who supported me regarding awards and promotions. I remembered hysterical Seattle travel stories with my work big brother, who always made me feel safe on the various planes, trains, and way too big SUVs. I even remembered seasoned teachers and administrators helping me along the way early in my K12 career.

Those people didn't take pity on me. Those people knew I was competent. Here was my perspective shift away from thinking I was a terrible decision-maker.

NO ONE ELSE saw me as defective and unable to make good decisions.

I was rewarded for consistently making good decisions.

After twenty-five years of carrying the belief that I couldn't make a good decision to save my life because of trusting my father when I was a teenager, I released that belief! The medicine allowed me to view my past differently and *see* that I had been a good decision maker my entire adult life!

It was clear that my father's actions were his and that he was a little child with layers. I didn't forgive him; I simply understood that part of my history from another perspective. I had done the work to release my trapped emotions from that night in my mother's apartment so that they no longer held any power. Yeah, it was shitty that it happened, but my flagellation from that night when I was sixteen was over.

Sixteen-year-old Jill would really be impressed by fifty-year-old Jill. Life turned out surprisingly good. I learned I didn't need to keep toxic people in my life. Sometimes I had to tolerate them at work, but I didn't invest emotionally in them. I didn't give any of myself to people who weren't worthy. The point is that my parents fucked up badly in taking care of me. That is the point. They didn't consider my future that day when THEY couldn't figure out a way to move forward in each other's lives. I could have been the most obedient or disobedient child, AND IT WOULD NOT HAVE MATTERED. My father would create chaos, and my mother was an emotional lightweight that couldn't model fighting him off. Their behavior was not because of me.

Trauma is highly personal, and I know my friends would have waved me off if I had shared my trapped feelings about that night when I was sixteen. Obviously, I couldn't *control* my parents, and my father's track record of chaos and destruction was his doing. I can't stress enough how the MDMA allowed me to process this information. Before the MDMA, my beliefs about that night were solid and trapped in my brain. I don't think any amount of talk therapy would have dislodged what I knew to be true—that I had fucked up big when I was sixteen.

So here I was, just one week out from my second

MDMA journey, and I felt lighter. I knew I didn't fuck up my life back then. I could suddenly appreciate just how un-fucked up my adult life had been with lots of excellent decisions.

I had some questions for my guides, though. I was a little confused about why I had spent time after both of my journeys on this trauma. Why did the medicine take me back to the same issue twice? Was there anything wrong with my brain that I couldn't make this perspective shift the first time around?

When we had our first post-journey talk therapy session, they assured me that nothing was wrong with my brain and that my healing was on track. It was common for PTSD patients to require multiple exposures to MDMA to unravel all the trapped emotions from their traumas. In fact, they encouraged me to review memories as much as I wanted in my journals. They emphasized that the healing journey would be an unraveling of memories at my brain's pace.

The more we talked, the more I thought about the process of cleaning a grimy frying pan. I could see the MDMA being the dish soap, while my integration was how I scrubbed the pan. So, after the first journey, the *At Sixteen I Fucked Up* pan was a little cleaner after a few bits and pieces of my trauma were released. But there was still a good amount of grime left that needed another journey. The second dose of MDMA gave me more dish soap, and I scrubbed away the rest of that grime very quickly into my integration.

I used that cleaning dirty pots imagery in my journals to give myself grace around the digital acres of repetitive writing. To me, all that writing told me my brain was healing a trauma point. I gave my fingers permission to kick the shit out of my laptop keyboard and write as much as I wanted, anytime I wanted, so I could keep cleaning.

Chapter 31

Second Place

While the early part of my second integration work focused on my fears, I transitioned into memories that pointed to my "stop feeling I'm not good enough" intention during the second week of my integration.

Over a week, my inner voice chatted about some memories while I walked Sadie. Individually, they seemed irrelevant, but together they showed me how I learned to think of myself. Thank goodness I journaled because the memories came to me at various times. If I hadn't journaled, I'm not sure I would have seen their impact on my psyche.

The memories that surfaced were those where I felt PTSD symptoms. I had interesting dog walks where some of those memories made my stomach twist, my throat tighten like I was ready to vomit, or red-hot anger surged through my shoulders. I was surprised at how quickly my body's reactions mirrored my memories so well. I thought I was getting better at this integration stuff because I quickly accessed those childhood feelings with the memories. I couldn't remember much more than the skeletal parts of the memories, but the body sensations came immediately.

●●●●●●●

When I was maybe eight, my father and I lived with his girlfriend and her daughter. Even though they weren't married, I've always

136

thought of my older roller-skating buddy as my stepsister. We didn't live together for very long, but we had the classic sibling love/hate kind of relationship that makes us laugh now.

It must have been a holiday because we both got bikes one year. My father put together my stepsister's bike first and then worked on mine. I got to ride her bike, but I scratched it during my terrible braking attempt that drove me into some steps. My stomach sank when I saw my father's fury. I remember getting off the bike, trying to shrink and hide my tears as much as possible to avoid getting hit. I had to hear the vitriol about how stupid and uncoordinated I was. Just the memory of that public shaming in the driveway made my cheeks flame. Too many neighbors were out and about. I didn't get hit, but I felt that embarrassment as clearly at age fifty as I did at age eight. All because of a small scratch in the paint.

I remembered, even at that age, I thought, "Why does everything end in yelling and screaming?"

Then my memory shifted to the infamous report card incident. My fifth grade A's weren't "as valuable" as my stepsisters' sixth grade A's. She argued for, and got, more allowance than I. This was a home run in our sibling rivalry game. But the white-hot anger that ran through me, made me scowl. My stepsister got what she wanted from my father *easy peasy lemon squeezy* while I was routinely insulted and battered. The message was clear: I was never going to be good enough—nothing was fair—I was always going to be second.

Then "the playground interrogation" memories showed up. My father couldn't abuse/hit anyone else in the house, so I got the brunt of his frustration. His tall frame towered over me while he asked about thirty "why" questions. He would ask, "Why did you go to the playground? Why did you stay at the playground? Why did you play at the playground?" I frantically tried to answer "correctly" to avoid getting slapped after each "wrong" answer. Those interrogations were his way to batter me a few times a month when no one else was in the house, in between more oversized fits of anger.

●●●●●●●

But then my stomach clenched hard, and I felt tears coming on. I pulled my baseball cap a little further down to hide my emotions from fellow dog walkers. I knew a challenging memory was next.

●●●●●●●

Their relationship imploded after my father and his girlfriend lived together for about two years. I was around ten at the time, so I don't know what happened, but I know I got blamed for it. My memory of that night started with me getting beaten in the downstairs bathroom. I was seated on the closed toilet. I sat there with my arms up, trying to protect myself as my father used me a punching bag.

Out of the corner of my eye, I saw my father's girlfriend dragging her daughter behind her as she scrambled past the bathroom door. She left the house because not soon after, my father pulled me out of the bathroom by my arm and threw me out the front door into the snow.

Her car was not in the driveway.

I wasn't surprised she left since she was the one who bought me long sleeve clothing to cover my bruises. She wasn't someone who expressed an interest in helping me.

So, there I was, without a coat in the Pennsylvania winter chill and a few inches of snow. I didn't know what to do. I walked to the side of the house to get out of the wind and just stood there. I didn't even go to a neighbor's house. I was ashamed, and I honestly didn't believe anyone would help. I wasn't worth anyone helping me. My stomach dropped when that feeling of worthlessness floated into focus.

I don't know how long I was out there until I heard the garage door open. My father came out, with his coat on, holding an ax. It still

**makes my throat tighten to remember how
ashamed I was that I wouldn't go to a
neighbor's house. I stood in the snow, skin
turning pink with cold, and watched that
monster yield an ax in front of me while I
waited for my mother to come. He had at least
called her—he wanted to be rid of me.**

●●●●●●●

I brushed away tears as Sadie and I reached the top of the
hill. Then I heard:

> **Inner Voice:** You learned you were second. You
> were taught other things, and people came in front
> of you. You don't even realize you believe it.

Second.
It didn't seem a particularly cruel word. It defined that
my wants and needs were not first to anyone. Not even
myself, as I learned early to regulate my emotions co-
dependently. The more I controlled my emotional
responses, the more I avoided the random verbal and
physical abuse that punctuated my childhood.

Then as Sadie and I finally got home, I remembered my
first year of teaching. That memory seemed out of place
with those other childhood memories, but I let it play out.

●●●●●●●

**During my first year of teaching, I
remembered getting a call in the office from a**

Delaware police officer because my mother had overdosed again. One of the student workers was concerned as I hung up the phone because she said she had never seen anyone sadder. I shrugged with defeat because that was my life. Even my need to focus on my fledgling career and a living wage job was second to dealing with my mother's neediness. My mother *tried* suicide about ten separate times throughout her life.

●●●●●●●

The integration's focus on these memories made me realize I always felt second or at least not first with either parent well into adulthood. If I always felt second, that meant that I never felt first.

I never voiced that feeling, but it was there all the time. Even one of the men I dated after Carl's death commented on how accommodating I was to his interests. I was just so used to going with the flow, and I never expressed myself when I sat at endless date night beer tastings when I hated beer.

Feeling second also made much of my success bittersweet. I smiled and accepted kudos throughout my career, and none of those achievements came close to erasing that worthless feeling. I didn't know how to feel proud of anything because I had a deep knowledge that I wasn't worth being in the spotlight. I had honed some ninja-level codependency skills to survive and accepted my *place* with people.

Even one of my managers once noticed my discomfort with my success. She encouraged me to enjoy the attention of a big award while I had it. While I was impressed with her insight, I couldn't follow her advice. I didn't know how to be first.

This integration work was massive. I would never have created a detective "crazy wall" that connected those memories before. It was only by reading my journals and seeing these particular memories strung together that I got it. I wish I understood exactly how this happened, but at the end of the day, I had to chalk it up to the power of the medicine. I finally had a reason why I assumed everything else came before me. I would never have figured it out if my integration and journaling hadn't linked those dusty memories together.

This was the first step in changing how I felt about my place in the world and no longer feeling my stomach clench when I won awards or got recognition. I was long overdue to feel comfortable putting myself first.

Chapter 32

My Future's Color

Around three weeks into my integration, I had a *duh* moment. It was almost hidden in the pages and pages of my digital journals, but there is something to be said for capturing as many thoughts as possible.

I am extremely careful about my social media diet. The same way I don't cook bacon naked is the same way I protect myself from unrealistic or sensationalist Instagram accounts. It has always been important to carefully curate my scrolling dopamine drips with inspirational quotes, psychedelic research, trauma healing advice, and silly parrot parents showcasing "Wet Chicken Wednesdays." I've learned to feed my brain with positive and fun content, and I embarrassingly follow too many cheeky parrot accounts.

In November, a month before the second journey, I saw a post asking viewers about their futures' colors. I journaled about my concern since I saw my future as pure empty darkness. In some ways, that simple exercise explained why I pursued this therapy. I didn't see any future, let alone a happy one for myself.

If there is no future, then there is very little reason to live.

That was why my journey intention to get rid of my fear of the future was so important. I lived life on autopilot according to how I was supposed to live to stay safe. I needed to nurture my promising career and be careful with my finances. I did those things while I held my breath and waited for something awful to happen. I came to this

143

therapy primarily living on fear. It was exhausting.

I journaled and deep-dived into my life's choices. I wrote incessantly about my financial decisions, why I didn't have children, Carl, and all my career moves. My journals resembled another detective story's crazy wall of evidence. It took a good bit of review to catch the little hints buried throughout my writing. Then I had a *duh* moment!

I didn't have a crystal ball for any of the decisions I had made in life

I didn't know the future or the results my choices would bring when I made them.

I've made some fucking awesome decisions that have left me with wonderful memories of my life with Carl.

However, my journaling and *duh* moment didn't seem that powerful to me. I think because I was looking at the past. I didn't equate yet that since I had made some great choices, I would continue to make great choices and have a happy future. I just kept journaling, journaling, and doing more journaling about the past.

Then one night, the *duh* turned into a lightbulb moment. During dinner, my boyfriend and I talked about career changes and where we might relocate if a job offer was good enough. As we were chatting about cities, I suddenly remembered that Instagram question. I asked what color he saw his future—and he immediately said blue—like the sky. I smiled because that was a cool answer. Then I sat back and thought about the question for myself. I smiled even more when I told him my future was a mix of hazy pastels that didn't feel empty. I couldn't feel anything specific; I just noticed that I didn't have that empty *blah* feeling anymore.

Here we were, talking about *future* career changes and relocations, and *I wasn't terrified.*

This shift appeared tiny but was monumental. My writing about decisions and choices I made after I was nineteen seemed to re-wire my brain. I think the repetition (and boy did I write the same shit on different days) let me believe that the last twenty-five years were proof that life was good and that I had a future. I could trust that *the universe* would let me have a future without ripping it out from under me, like how it had happened so often when I was a child. It was like the medicine and integration process let me finally see the last twenty-five years instead of only looking at my life before I was twenty.

There were way too many exclamation marks when I wrote about those hazy pastels in my journal. I was excited because I saw specific proof that this therapy was making progress on that huge intention about the future. I mean, it was fine that I shifted my perspectives about my parents, but to see the shift in thinking about my future while it happened was remarkable.

Chapter 33

My Fashionista Flag

I know social media gets a bad rap, but I found a few Instagram accounts focused on trauma awareness to be incredibly helpful as I developed a language around my own healing. Dr. Nicole LePera and Nate Postlethwait run informative trauma accounts and have taught me about mental health and healing from bite-sized posts. I enjoyed being connected to online communities focused on improving mental health.

It was also from an Instagram post that I realized that I had all the adult warning signs of children who hadn't been able to express emotions. Low self-esteem, extreme worry, and a general lack of trust were the traits with which I most identified. As I did more research, I learned that codependency, in my non-doctor terms, was when I knew I was going to be ok when my parents were calm. Conversely, I was on thin ice when either parent was stressed. I learned to adapt to my parents' emotions and suppress mine as much as possible to avoid fights and my father's favorite non-bruising abuse, slapping me across the face.

As I read more, I realized my stellar ability to *read the room* and *raise people's energy* were just codependent behaviors I learned at an early age to keep myself safe.

I never learned to express my emotions, especially anger or fear, because there was no room for my emotions in my parents' lives. I believed, and was probably right, that expressing any anger or frustration would grow slaps into punches or get me thrown out of a house. Instead of paying attention to how I felt, I paid attention to how the person, or people I was living with, felt. More importantly, I paid awfully close attention to how they felt about me.

I realized I took responsibility for other people's emotions and even thoughts. I had a mental formula: "Jill does X, and it makes someone think or do Y." Consequently, I spent my whole life not trying to ruffle feathers or bring a lot of attention to myself.

When I realized from my Instagram scrolling where some of my behavior came from, I felt a sense of relief. Putting everyone else first was a learned behavior. It wasn't *how things are*.

So, it was interesting to see when the medicine allowed me to make a codependent shift in my thinking. Score one for journaling because I might have missed this breakthrough if I hadn't written about it.

My journal mentioned a quick reference to the Tuesday night routine at my boyfriend's place. It was our thing to grab some take-out, zone out, and watch stupid celebrity television. One Tuesday, I let my fashionista flag fly and gave my commentary on the celebrities' wardrobe choices. It was fun to unleash my snark for the denim puffed sleeve shirt aberration and the neon green glasses that had to have been at the bottom of the stylist's barrel. My boyfriend laughed right along with me because I couldn't stop with just one comment when the glitter headband made its way to the screen.

And I realized, as I let my snark shine, that my behavior was completely different from when we first met. In the beginning, I worked extremely hard to figure him out and see what made him laugh and smile. The irony was that he didn't wear his thoughts or feelings on his face. He is a super chill guy who thinks before he speaks. So, I got frustrated when I tried to understand where I would fit in with his interests and likes. My codependency skills hit a brick wall with him.

Ultimately, I couldn't suppress my wit as I began to trust him. Wackiness routinely tumbled out of my mouth. I learned I couldn't completely change who I was, and he wasn't there for a mirror. He enjoyed my energy.

That night marked an important milestone for me, though. I showed my opinion and expressed my fashion commentary that usually stayed in my head. I stopped being concerned that my boyfriend would not be happy with me since I could be *mean* while expressing my inner Joan Rivers. I was fashion judgmental! It was so much fun and harmless, but I had yet to show that side of me for fear of being labeled *mean*.

Something so little, yet significant, was a step out of codependency. Letting my stream of consciousness flow without restraint was freeing, and I enjoyed being seen for who I was.

I hadn't done that since Carl died. He was the only person who knew me unfiltered.

Through reading about MDMA, I learned that the drug made users more empathic to themselves. I completely believe MDMA let me be kinder to myself. I had finally made the first step to feeling *it is ok to be Jill* in a few situations. This is an excellent example of a small integration step that was an unexpected breakthrough.

I look at it this way: at least there was a practical use for the denim, 1980s acid-washed top with puffy sleeves.

Chapter 34

Empathy, Not Forgiveness

A month after my second journey, my father was disproportionately in my head. I'm not proud of that, but it would have been a short book if I glossed over the process and pretended to send all the years of negativity and abuse to voicemail. My journals had tornadoes of thought like the tornadoes I wrote the previous week. They swirled and spiraled with stories about my father's abuse. The medicine had shown me I still had tons of trapped emotions around my father, and I needed to address them. The repetition was my step-by-step healing as I understood that my father's behavior was not my fault. He was someone deeply haunted.

Then one Saturday, I had a very tough day. I was doing everyday chores and had the TV on in the background for noise. There was a crime show with a scene in a mental institution where a female patient got visibly upset during a visit from her abuser. As with all crime dramas that need to move fast, the detectives were in the right place, at the right time, and saw the interaction. The victim had never told anyone that this man had hurt her. In what the abuser thought was a private conversation, he threatened and insulted the victim while she crossed her arms in front of her for a semblance of protection.

I remember the female detective pointing out that the abuser had let his guard down when he didn't realize he was being observed. He had turned into Mr. Hyde right in front of the two-way mirror.

That line stopped me. I felt my chest get tight like I was suffocating. I remember I had to consciously work on my breathing.

Then a deeply buried memory floated into focus:

●●●●●●●

When I was a senior in high school, I was in a bad car accident. I was a new driver and made a rookie mistake that totaled my father's car. Luckily, everyone walked away with only bruises.

I was absolutely terrified of my father's reaction and was genuinely frightened at how he would react. Even then I knew that money was far more important to him than I was.

I was surprised when he showed up on the scene and was calm when he talked to the officers. I'm sure he spoke to me, but I don't remember it. I only remember how charming and relaxed he seemed while at the accident scene when he spoke to the police and emergency services folks. Only I knew the show he was performing. He had perfected being charming and polite in his various sales jobs.

I remember vividly how he treated me after we left the scene. For some reason, we walked back to his apartment and when the streets were empty, he would slap or punch me. I was already bruised from the accident so a few more bruises wouldn't raise any alarms. He made me walk in front of him so I didn't exactly know when I would get hit. And

150

while I don't remember most of his yelling, I remember that he called me a *fucking cunt* a few times. It was hard to miss as the insults were timed when he would hit me and sometimes knock me into the street.

●●●●●●●

I have never been called a cunt by any other person. He holds that award.

By this point, I had sat down to catch my breath and think about this memory. I had learned by then that going toward the uncomfortable was the way to heal.

I realized his behavior was the textbook opposite of what to do when someone has had a traumatic experience like a car accident. Slapping, hitting, and cursing as we walked to his apartment certainly was not the way to treat a child. But I wondered why this memory came up, right now, at this moment.

Then I realized this memory was triggered by the Mr. Hyde comment on the TV show.

The MDMA had been allowing me to see my parents differently. They had their own traumas and I was slowly, with lots of journal writing, reframing my internal narrative that something about me caused them to treat me as they did. I also had more empathy for them because, from my adult perspective, I could see how unhappy their lives were.

But I think my mind needed to remind me that my father's abusive behavior wasn't just a simple result of his trauma. He was a monster who could control his behavior and emotions. He controlled his emotions and was charming in front of the police at the accident, with family, and with women in the early dating stages until they figured out he was all smoke and mirrors.

He chose violence and cruelty towards my mother and me *when no one could see it.* He knew hurting us was wrong. He chose violence anyway.

My father certainly deserved empathy for whatever trauma haunted him, but he was responsible for his atrocious behavior.

He didn't deserve my forgiveness.

Chapter 35

I Deserve a Future

Most of my integration's perception shifts happened gradually by writing in my journal. Looking back now, I can see how it took days and weeks for me to shift my feelings and ideas around my childhood memories.

But there were other points in my integration where my perspective shifts came *at* me instead. Usually, I would be doing something mindless, like walking Sadie or unloading the dishwasher, and suddenly an emotion or memory would crash into me like a giant ocean wave. It was similar to how I sometimes experienced unexpected waves of grief that almost knocked me over after Carl's death. My mind and body would fill with extreme anger or sadness that usually brought me to tears at unexpected times.

During integration, emotional outbursts didn't happen often. But when they came, they forced me to listen!

I wrote about an afternoon of mundane chores. In mid-towel-fold, I yelled, "I DESERVE A FUTURE. I DESERVE A FUTURE." My throat was tight, and I had to sit down on the floor. I even wondered if I was having a mini-panic attack. I remember Sadie trotted over to see what the drama was about. She looked at me, head sideways, and her cuteness stopped my frustrated yelling.

I felt distraught and lost. I started to dry heave through tears while I focused on Sadie to try and calm down. I repeated, "I deserve a future" a few times until I calmed down and said it in a whisper.

Sadie did her job and curled next to me while I caught

my breath. My mind went back to my mom's apartment after she slapped me when I was sixteen. That was the first time my mother had recycled my father's favorite way to humiliate us. If there was one thing I could have screamed, it would have been, "I deserve a future!" I've always thought that my parents' decisions that day were to try and STOP my future from being good. I took their actions that personally.

They didn't see it that way. They probably didn't do it on purpose. I don't think they understood the ramifications of their actions short or long term. Neither of them had gone to college and didn't understand scholarships. But to me, at the time, they were stopping my future. They didn't realize it, but from that moment forward, I shut them out of knowing who I was for the rest of their lives. I never let them hear my hopes and dreams.

I couldn't trust them.

By the end of my outburst, I felt so much better. With Sadie earning a bonus snack for doing her doggie cuddling job well, I went back to folding the towels. I grinned at my freedom to yell and scream in my own house whenever I wanted. I felt lighter after my outburst.

I smiled as I realized I hadn't trusted my parents my entire adult life and, consequently, *neither* had derailed my lovely long-term relationship with Carl or my career. I think I needed to be reminded that I had managed to keep both at arm's length and that I *had* created a great life without them.

Later that day I wrote:

> *Wow. There is quite a bit of emotion there. And*
> *anger. I have no idea if I ever dealt with that anger*
> *towards them. I don't remember doing so. It was*

much more of a withdrawal. These people were dangerous, and they would stay at arm's reach. They weren't going to get to know me so they could stop me in other ways.

At that moment, at sixteen, I stopped trying beyond the basics with them. Even when mom took me back in, I didn't share my thoughts and feelings with her. I didn't share my life in any detail. My mom and I didn't have the "give me a call every week" type of relationship. We could easily go a few months without connecting. And as soon as I could create boundaries to get my father out of my life—I did.

I wasn't ever going to let them get close enough to stop my future.

Chapter 36

The Nightmare

A few months after my second journey, in early March, I was chatting with a friend who also carried childhood trauma. He was further down the healing road than I, and he talked about healing his core wound. We both understood that core wounds are deep wounds that subconsciously impact our adult lives. Our chat was almost prescient as I started dealing with a terrible nightmare that I couldn't shake by the end of March. It stayed with me like it was glued behind my eyes.

In my nightmare, I saw myself at five, with a child's body and monster head. It wasn't a very creative monster head. As a child of the 1980s, my head happened to look like a Pacman circle with massive teeth. Seriously! I was a little girl with a black Pacman-like, eyeless face with a wide mouth of shark-layered teeth. I wore a simple black dress, white stockings, and little Mary Jane shoes. I was downstairs in my childhood house in the front room (where the door to the house had been), and I was crouched downstairs, by the staircase, like a frightened animal with my jaws chomping.

I woke from that nightmare in a cold sweat. I wouldn't say I liked dreaming of my childhood house, which I always just called by its street name, Lanner Street. Also, I wouldn't say I liked the trapped feeling that weighed down my body. I felt that little girl's intense fear and wanted to protect her from some unseen danger.

But she couldn't escape. She needed those fierce teeth for

protection.

I scheduled a chat with my therapist, and we talked about this nightmare and how I couldn't shake this feeling that something out *there* was dangerous. I couldn't define the *there* or the *what* that was dangerous. I just knew something big could go bad soon, and I would have to fight to survive.

With my therapist's gentle questioning, I shaped that little girl monster into what I remember I looked like when I was five. I was a tad tall for my age, slim, had very light brown hair that curled at my neck, and my adult teeth were just starting to come in haphazardly since I had knocked out my two front baby teeth with a clumsy fall in the driveway. At my therapist's advice, over the next few weeks, I meditated by visiting that little girl at Lanner Street. We both believed that little girl was trying to tell us something.

Eventually, in my meditations, I was able to get little Jill a comfortable pink nightgown and matching fuzzy slippers. When I pictured the room, I had redecorated it. I couldn't actually remember what that room really looked like, so it was easy to turn it into a lovely bedroom filled with toys, warm clothes, and a bed covered by a fluffy comforter designed for snuggling.

It got to the point in my meditations that I read to this Jill, and she fell asleep cushioned by a mountain of plush pillows.

But there was no way out. There was no door to Lanner Street. I couldn't get that Jill to even go near the wall where that door had been in real life.

That was the vital part of my meditations that confused me. I thought the point of my meditations was to get my little self out of that house. That was the house where my father beat us, and my mother tried to kill herself countless times. That was the staircase my father had thrown me down and then thrown me around the room. This is the room where I had huddled while my mother screamed while my father beat her.

I thought it was apparent that I needed to get that little girl out!

When I tell this story, what people find interesting, and what I found maddening at the time, was that little Jill didn't want to leave Lanner Street during my meditations. How could she not want to leave that house of horrors? How could she not see that a safe adult would walk her out of that horrible house? What was I missing? At one point, I even thought I was meditating wrong because when I approached little Jill with curiosity about why she wouldn't leave, she wouldn't say. Because she was quiet, I assumed this was about fear of the future, and she was terrified that anything outside of the house could be worse than the lovely little bedroom I had created for her. And by the way, the staircase to the room had been sealed off. No one could get into that room and hurt her. I guessed she was safe for the first time in her life and was happy to stay that way.

As my therapist and I worked for weeks on this mental puzzle, I could feel the stress in my body. I didn't sleep well, and my neck was constantly burning with an odd sense of fear. That little girl was always in the back of my mind. We finally admitted that learning what kept little Jill in that horrible house couldn't be accessed by my conscious mind.

We scheduled my third journey for late May.

Chapter 37

Transcripts Ahead

I was glad we could schedule my third journey for the end of May. It coincided with my birthday, and I used the journey as an excuse to take a few vacation days to celebrate making it through another year. I also wanted to give my brain integration time and have the luxury of stopping to journal whenever I wanted.

That journey's central theme, or intention, was to get that five-year-old Jill out of Lanner Street. I didn't know why it was so important, only that it was. My subconscious dropped breadcrumbs that I had a much larger issue to deal with when I dreamed of myself with a monster's head back in March. My therapist and I hadn't been successful in freeing that little girl with our talk therapy sessions, and I felt that her freedom was vitally important. I didn't know why it was so important, but that nightmare clarified that something in my subconscious wanted to be brought to my conscious mind. So, that intention was front and center.

I still had bits and pieces of being scared about the future and feeling like the universe was against me. But that little Jill, unable to leave that house, which had been full of pain and abuse, couldn't be ignored.

When we all met in mid-May for our pre-journey talk therapy session, I reviewed my intentions. My guide gently suggested that we consider adding psilocybin (magic mushrooms) to the journey since so little progress in freeing little Jill had been made through our months of talk therapy. I don't recall the specifics of our conversation after that because all I remember was my sense of relief. My guides had a plan. I felt like I had been holding my breath for months, and I could finally exhale.

The healing from my two prior MDMA journeys happened with perspective shifts during my integration phases. My journals during those integrations detailed my mental gymnastics of how I looked at my childhood differently, with empathy, and released so much fear and shame. The months of my integrations were full of diving into harrowing childhood memories and cleansing them of the mental and physical power they held over me.

The third journey didn't follow that same pattern. During my third journey, with MDMA and then psilocybin, the most profound healing happened *while* I was medicated, and there was little integration compared to the first MDMA-only journeys. So, I decided to share about 15% of the transcripts and memories from that day because they were so powerful. After my third journey, I was a different person inside. I no longer had a ball of fear that sat in my chest that I had carried for decades. I only knew the weight of that ball of fear when it was lifted off me during that third journey.

I hope sharing some of the transcripts will show how my subconscious fought to keep me safe and how the medicine won against my trapped emotions that dripped with fear from when I was five. Sharing these transcripts has been profoundly personal, so I only selected the portions I thought showed the most healing progress. Since my goal with this book was to explain, to the best of my ability, how psychedelic-assisted psychotherapy can work, I thought it necessary to include relevant transcripts to shine a light on the moments of healing with these medications.

My third journey's conversation kept going back to self-worth like my first two journeys, but I'll admit I got tired of reading the repetitive parts of the transcripts. I was kind of over the fact that I wasn't over that shit. Consequently, I didn't include those parts of the transcript because I get it; after a while, it gets old! The rest of the boring, repetitive transcripts that could put a caffeinated toddler to sleep are safely tucked away in my journals.

I mention my repetition to normalize trauma patients' needs to keep unraveling their trapped emotions around trauma, layer by layer. Thankfully, my digital journal never charged by the page because I had so many stories and ideas repeated until they held no emotional or physical power over me.

Since my goal has been to describe how my psychedelic-assisted psychotherapy worked, I think the following segments spotlight what skilled guides, psychedelics, and a willing patient can do to heal childhood trauma-induced PTSD.

I invite you to come along with me as I healed a major core wound from my childhood and shifted my entire perspective about my place in the world. Finally, the title of this book will make sense!

Chapter 38

My Third Journey

At the end of May, my third journey again started in the beautiful healing room. I had been encouraged to bring anything that would help me focus on my intentions. In the past two journeys, I had pushed back against that advice because I didn't want to be a bother. I don't know how bringing something to my journey would be considered a bother, but that was how my mind thought before. I was extremely comfortable this time and decided to bring a small poster taken from my living room wall.

A few months prior, I grabbed a meme from the Internet of a little girl in a bathing suit who seemed to be belting out a primal roar in the rain. I turned that meme into a poster because that picture depicts the pure joy of a girl not being afraid one bit of being who she is. That little girl hadn't had layers of conformity from society, parents, or even school piled on her yet. Most importantly, she wasn't a victim of abuse.

The meme's caption said: *She is still there...inside you... waiting. Let's go get her.*

That picture not only aligned with my intention to free that five-year-old from Lanner Street, but it succinctly described the work my guides and I had to do. Freeing her wouldn't be easy; we had to rescue her.

After the three of us settled in the sitting area I described why I had brought my poster. My therapist had a lovely surprise. She gave me a little orange and white Tigger stuffed animal from Winnie the Pooh. In some random conversation about fearing my father, I told her how when I was eight, I started to hide my Tigger in a closet every day before school, so my father couldn't hurt him or take him away. I had very few childhood things because I had moved so much, but I managed to keep Tigger with me. But when my father threw me out of his house when I was ten, I couldn't grab that little stuffed tiger whose right leg was attached by my crisscrossed, uneven, red stitches.

Getting that stuffed animal from my therapist was a sign for me. It was ok to go back to the memories of when I was five. My guides weren't going to be mean or, even worse, laugh at my pain. They weren't getting frustrated that I wasn't over my shit. (I was super frustrated because I am the most impatient person I have ever met.). Instead, that little stuffed toy gave me the message—it was ok to visit and hang out with five-year-old Jill. That little tiger was both an invitation and the acceptance from my guides that I could visit my inner five-year-old, and they would be there to keep me safe.

At that point, I took the MDMA capsules since we were all clear on the intentions for the day. Then my guide started chatting about the concept of childhood-created avatars. He explained that children make avatars, or ways to think about themselves, to survive abuse. These avatars can take any shape and have any meaning. I remember thinking, "Oh, he gets it," because for most of my life, when things got tough, my back would straighten up, and I would get very still because I felt strength run through my back. That steel I envisioned that ran the length of my back was there to keep me standing against anything that came my way. I used to explain it by my philosophy, "quiet confidence always wins," because whenever I felt threatened and sat up straight, I tended to slow down and became hyper-vigilant. Acrimonious budget meetings, coworkers causing chaos, prickly customers, and stressful career events made me straighten my back and speak very carefully. While I radiated active listening and confidence, inside I braced for attacks.

As the MDMA entered my system, I described my avatar. It was like a steel rod that supported my body. It allowed me to stand straight; it held me up when I was scared, exhausted, or sad. When things got bad, that internal steel rod said:

This is going to suck.

Get ready for the suck.

I'm going to get you through the suck.

It kept my back straight and shoulders tensed as I battled any perceived threat.

That steel rod refused more beatings when I was nineteen. That steel rod worked two jobs while going to college. That steel rod excised my father from most of my adult life. That steel rod took over during job interviews. That steel rod was my invisible partner-in-crime that allowed me to function in what my inner child knew was a dangerous world.

That steel rod stopped me from taking my life to join Carl after he passed.

That steel rod that ran down my back had an unwavering focus on survival. That shiny, strong, childhood-created avatar could turn into a sword when I felt things were getting too out of control. I could be viciously judgmental, intimidatingly assertive, and even cruel. Anything that seemed to vaguely, and I mean vaguely, threaten me financially (aka the work drama created from a coworker's shenanigans and my email response) brought out that steel rod that could become a vicious verbal sword that, when used, often created awkward silences as people searched to lessen the tension in the room. I didn't use that sword often, but when I did, I felt terrible about those interactions.

What I missed, and my guides didn't, was that my steel rod was just one of my avatars. Little Healthy Jill, the little five-year-old child who wouldn't leave that awful house, who first showed herself to me as a little monster with razor-sharp teeth to defend herself—she was an avatar! I wrote in my journal:

> *She was that little girl who didn't help her mother during my father's beatings.*
> *She was the little girl whose basic instinct to survive made her huddle downstairs while hearing her mother's cries.*
> *She was the little girl who knew she was a cold, mean person who didn't deserve love.*

My guides knew that even though she now looked like an average five-year-old in my mind, she, herself, was an avatar for a terrified Jill somewhere trapped in Lanner Street.

Chapter 39

Malnourished Jill

Our conversation about avatars lasted until the MDMA started to take effect. As we all moved to the other side of the room so I could lie down, we had a fantastic discovery.

Guide: Can we check in with the little girl on Lanner Street?
Jill: Well, we are with Jill downstairs. Upstairs Jill is trapped. She is Stressed Jill. Downstairs Jill is fun Jill. Downstairs Jill is jumping up and down.

And there it was. *Upstairs Jill is trapped. She is Stressed Jill.*

There was a five-year-old Jill, upstairs in her childhood room, who was stressed. My conscious mind didn't know about that five-year-old Stressed Jill. My guides told me later they had known for weeks that Downstairs Jill was an avatar. After all, I had tried to get Little Jill, or Downstairs Jill, out of that house for months. She wouldn't budge.

The whole time, there was a little girl upstairs who couldn't get out of Lanner Street too. My Downstairs Jill was *her* avatar to survive. It suddenly made sense why Downstairs Jill never saw a door to leave that house. Upstairs Jill couldn't leave her room.

This breakthrough showed the sheer power of MDMA and trusted guides. It allowed me to get to what I can only call my core mental injury that needed healing. That Upstairs Jill was the Jill who knew in her bones *there was no way out* and *there was no future* and she would always be alone, trapped in her childhood bedroom.

Can you blame her? Her life consisted of her childhood room, upstairs in that awful house next to her parents' bedroom where she could hear her father beating her mother at night. She *knew* there wasn't anything good on the other side of her bedroom door.

Chapter 40

Stealthy Jill

My guides noted the second Jill in the upstairs room, but they didn't push me to talk about her so early in the journey. Instead, we talked more about Downstairs Jill as an avatar. We also talked about my overall competency and internal drive.

One of the weirdest challenges of my childhood was that I was expected to succeed, but my father wasted no opportunity to tell me how ugly and stupid I was. That kind of abuse escalated in proportion to my achievements. I learned to hide my accomplishments as much as possible, and I took that habit into adulthood. I don't know when I first learned this lesson, but I was a bright kid who did well in school, so I think I learned it early in my life.

Instead of understanding that my father was just an asshole who couldn't be happy for anyone else, my child-centric mind interpreted that I couldn't be too happy or proud because the universe wouldn't like it.

The result? It has been a lifetime of being too humble and keeping my head down below anyone's radar. It absolutely impacted my career. I couldn't own my strength and leadership even though my daily activities showed my innate power and leadership. I felt like a little kid, afraid to sit at the big people's table, but I was preparing and eating the same filet mignon on the folding chairs at the pop-up kids' table.

About ninety minutes into the MDMA session:

168

———

Guide: This is where I see this ancient, deep conditioning. Don't let it show. Terrible things will happen. Do whatever you have to do.

Therapist: This is definitely a relationship to your power that we are speaking to. There is a danger that if you show your power, you will come under attack. So, your power has to be masked. And you can't let it get to your highest potential because that will attract too much attention. Those are very, very old patterns, and they are in the way of you fully expressing who you are in the world. The gift that you are.

Jill: (Frustrated) Just the work it has taken to stealthily be me. Heavy. (Raised my hand to my upper chest.)

Guide: So, go towards that heaviness in your chest if you can. What is that thing on your chest right now?

Jill: (Pause) It stops me, it stops me from getting hit. (Sadly) That is what came to me.

Guide: So it is like armor that defends and protects you. But at the same time, it is heavy body armor. You have to walk with it. Let's get a feeling for the density of that body armor if you can. (Curious) Can you get a sense of how heavy that is?

Jill: It is constant work.

Guide: Does it feel like a material, like energy? What is this thing that is on you?

Jill: (Thinking pause) Ahh, very strong mesh to allow for a bit of leeway.

169

I started to talk about the heaviness of staying under the radar like an internal mesh running through me. It wasn't like screen mesh. It was more like the classic green wire fencing. When I was with other talented and quick-witted people, that mesh would allow more of me to show through. But when I was with my parents, it held me back so I wouldn't face criticism or physical abuse.

I mentioned that my parents didn't know me at all.

Guide: You can bring that as an inquiry for yourself. Cause you know, Upstairs Jill, deep down in that bunker (meaning the bunker of her upstairs room), she realized very quickly, these are not her people. She was told they were because they were her parents.

Jill: They are supposed to be my people.

Guide: They should be, but these are not your people. She knew as soon as she could—she needed an escape strategy. As soon as she got an opportunity, she got out of there.

Jill: Yes, regardless of how painful it was.

Guide: Could you get how brilliant and smart she was to survive all those years?

Jill: I don't take compliments well.

Guide: You don't have to. I am talking to *her* anyway. You want to let *her* get and recognize *her* brilliance. *She* knew these were not her people. *She* built this amazing avatar to protect her and survive. Stealth is not pretension. Stealth is brilliance.

Jill: She doesn't look brilliant. She seems close to

dying.

Guide: Can you describe her?

———————

The transcript got very choppy while I described that little girl stuck in her childhood room. In my mind, I could see that she was nothing like any childhood picture I have of myself. It was like a horror film director created a frightened Jill character. This Jill had a tiny, malnourished body and was dressed in a black romper from the 1970s. She had a large head with scraggly black hair that fell around her face because she was slumped protectively into herself. Her room only had a bed that looked like a white rectangular box without pillows, sheets, or blankets. I could see her sitting on the side of her bed in an empty, starkly white room that had the door to the hallway closed.

She looked dangerously malnourished. She sat there, head down, back hunched, and twirled her hair.

I used to twirl my hair right out of my head when I was that age.

I then took a little break during the journey and went quiet. I remember feeling an incredible sadness while I had described what I was now calling, Malnourished Jill. I needed to absorb that I had an inner child inside me that was so monumentally sad and frightened that she was withering away.

Chapter 41

I'm Not Good Enough

My guides gave me the quiet time I needed, and when I engaged with them again, they focused on my intention.

One thing about this medicine, and the immense trust I had in my guides, is that I could spill all the awful things that even taste foul when they come out of my mouth. The things I couldn't say in polite company were welcomed. The next portion of the journey shifted to some well-hidden feelings that I can't remember ever admitting before.

Guide: Let's go back to your little girl.

Jill: Which one? The one in the bad room or the good room?

Guide: Well, the question is to either one or both. What do they need so they can come out? What do they need from you so they can come out?

Jill: Hmmm. I need it to be safe. Jill in the good bedroom downstairs—I need it to be safe. I need it to be fun. There's gotta be someone to love. I'm kinda empty.

Guide: Someone to play with?

Jill: No. She wants to love somebody.

Guide: Someone to love?

Jill: She wants to love somebody. She didn't love them.

Guide: She didn't love her mom and dad. Got it.

Jill: She wanted their, you know, everything a child wants, approval. It was a constant fight for that. But I didn't really love them. I didn't love my mother. I'm not allowed to say that. I hoped that maybe if I did this or that or the other thing, it would be enough. Even up to folding her fucking clothes after she died, I hoped it would be enough.

————————

Not loving my parents, I thought, was a significant deficiency *in me*. I never loved them. In fact, I didn't really like them most of the time. I tolerated them and learned my codependent survival behaviors in response to their emotional deficiencies. I always wanted them to love me, to take care of me, and for me to experience the joy and cuddles those other kids got on TV. But the truth of the matter was, I was finally able to face the shame of my feelings about my parents during this journey. I didn't love them.

————————

Guide: Does Jill love herself?

Jill: No.

Guide: She doesn't love herself.

Jill: Because for so long she couldn't be who she was.

Guide: So, let's stay with this part a bit—that she doesn't love herself. What does she need to love herself?

Jill: (Dejected) She needed Carl. It was external.

———————

This was one of the times I gasped while listening to the transcript. I don't remember most of the journey, and to see myself saying that the only way I knew to love myself was through Carl's love was like a punch in the gut. It made sense, though; he was the first to love me unconditionally and where I felt loved.

———————

Guide: This part of you that doesn't love you, was that why you needed Carl? Is there some aspect in you that you don't love yourself? That you aren't deserving of love? Is there some message that you got from your parents that you are not lovable?

Jill: I'm not good enough. I will never be good enough.

Guide: So, I want to reframe that narrative. And the reframe is NOT that you are not good enough and are insufficient for anyone to love you. The reframe is that *they* just weren't capable of loving.

Jill: (Pause) I would agree with that.

Guide: Now use that reframe because you are holding on to another belief. You're taking it on as if you are at fault. "I was not lovable. I'm broken. That is why they didn't love me." And I'm saying, hold on, I'm not sure that is really how it went down. It just went that way because you happened to fall on…

Jill: Those two.

Guide: Part of your current journey in this life is that you needed to experience this somehow. They just weren't capable of loving.

Jill: No, they really weren't.

Guide: Yeah, they weren't. On the other hand, you are very capable of loving, as discovered with your relationship with Carl. Let's just come back to this aspect of not loving yourself. Is that reframe working?

Jill: Is it working?

Guide: In the sense of reframing this aspect that you don't love yourself?

Jill: (Hesitant) No. I don't know. When I love myself, I get too proud. I get too big for my britches. When I am proud of myself, I need something to tone it down. I can't get too big for my britches. I don't know where that comes from.

Guide: Do you want to go find out? Are you curious about that?

Jill: I have always been curious about that.

Guide: So, let's start this getting big. Imagine yourself getting as big as you can imagine yourself getting. Right. Go towards it. And see what wants to show up. What happens when you go toward it?

———————

I didn't go toward it. It was too scary. I just went quiet.

I remember being very frustrated when I transcribed the transcript that I didn't figure out why *getting big* and being proud of myself was so bad. I still didn't know exactly where the thought about being too big for my britches came from. While writing out the transcript, I hoped my integration process would delve into this trauma point at some point and help me uncover the origin of thinking I could possibly get *too big for my britches*.

175

Healing this "too big for my britches" trauma point took only a few weeks after the journey. One day I ran across this quote on Reddit, "When you're not used to being confident, confidence feels like arrogance."

I don't have many childhood positive experiences of getting feedback when I did something noteworthy (good grades, awards at school). I learned at an early age that succeeding and being proud of myself led to hurtful words and my father slapping me across the face. So, it made sense that my mind turned confidence into a harmful arrogance to avoid getting hurt. Unfortunately, since most adults are just little kids wrapped in adult layers, I continued to think confidence was bad into my adulthood. In fact, that entire thinking process around confidence and arrogance led to incredible amounts of imposter syndrome in my career.

Suddenly, like the quick double snaps I tend to do while teaching, I let the baggage I had been carrying about success and confidence go. I looked at my life differently and allowed myself to be proud of all I had achieved. It was finally ok to be proud of how I had lived my life. I had a successful career. I could look at my paid-off little condominium, which had been the home to several spoiled, happy pets, and be thankful for all the lovely memories embedded in its walls instead of thinking I didn't deserve the security of a house. Most importantly, I could be proud of being half of a loving, long-term relationship for twenty years.

●●●●●●●●

Chapter 42

She Does It to Herself

Since I shut down when I was asked to go towards *being bigger* in the world, my guides let me sit quietly. The medicine in my system was doing its job and highlighting childhood memories that applied to my intentions.

When I peeked my head up again, I talked about the struggle I felt about being successful at work and trying to dodge the spotlight. It was a weird way to live because tooting one's own horn is how careers progressed at my corporate job. If I did something great for a customer or the company, and no one in leadership knew about it, did it really happen?

My guides, who very often mirrored my conversation, asked me if my avoidance strategy had been working.

––––––––––

> **Jill:** Well, what's been good for me so far is hiding.
> **Guide:** Only as a strategy coming from believing that you need to fear the world.
> **Jill:** I would agree with you on that.
> **Guide:** That is the strategy of a very young child who needs to feel safe with you to come out into the world.
> **Jill:** Is that really what is holding Jill in? Is that really what is holding Jill in that fun, downstairs bedroom? Not so much that it is scary out there. That I will scare people away by being mean? I will have people do terrible things to me because I am

mean?

Guide: Who is saying that to you?

Jill: (Struggling) I don't know. That was hard to get to.

Guide: Take a look right there. Who is saying that to you? Who is saying that to the little girl?

Jill: What? That she will get hurt?

Guide: Yeah. Who is saying that to her?

Jill: Five-year-old Jill in the upstairs bedroom. She is twirling her hair on the side of the bed. That's who is saying it. That is exactly who is saying it.

Guide: What is happening is what I call an inside job. She is doing it.

Jill: Doing it to herself?

Guide: She is doing it to herself. What she has done is she has built this elaborate castle. She is on the inside. On the outside, she has put all these amazing avatars that allow her to succeed and survive the world. There is only one downside; to make her survive and succeed in the world, her avatars (Downstairs Jill, steel rod) are also her jailers. Because they are the ones who turn around to her and say, "You can't go out there, Jill, it is too dangerous. We need to keep you in here." It is not her dad; it is not her mom. They are long gone. Her avatars are both her protectors and her jailers. She put them out there to protect her. She wants to go out but like, no fucking way, it is too dangerous.

JILL: (Exasperated) My inner voice just said, "You had twenty-five years of proof it's not dangerous. Figure it out."

GUIDE: Yeah. It's not going to get figured out at this point. So, we're going to give you some

179

mushrooms.

_____

Chapter 43

No Trust

I wasn't ready for the mushrooms. I didn't know what they would do, but I felt they would be transformative. There was something scary about the *newness* of what my life would be like after healing. After all, I had never lived without my fear to guide and protect me. My guides always let me set the journey's pace, so they waited.

I'm not going to lie. The next phase of the journey was challenging for me, and the transcript shows my guides' patience because I rambled while I tried to get upstairs to help Malnourished Jill. I needed lots of pauses, and I could hear the sadness in my voice in the transcript. There was no reframing. This part of the journey was slowly uncovering the Malnourished Jill who had crouched like a frightened animal in my head for forty-five years.

My guides guided me by asking if I could get healthy Downstairs Jill to my upstairs childhood bedroom to meet Malnourished Jill.

When I was able to have them meet, it was a breakthrough!

●●●●●●●●

Malnourished Jill looked at her healthy avatar and drank in her age-appropriate size, healthy skin, and chubby cheeks. Downstairs Jill, in a sunny yellow baby doll dress, white stockings, and white patent leather shoes,

looked ready to go to a birthday party.

Malnourished Jill allowed Downstairs Jill to sit on the side of the bed next to her. Healthy Jill opened her arms for a hug, and Malnourished Jill folded under Downstairs Jill's shoulder and allowed herself to be cuddled. She didn't hug back, though; she could only receive caring. She was empty and didn't have anything to give.

●●●●●●●

It would be the classic "aww" moment in a movie when an older sister hugs a younger sister. But here they were, the same age, but they had just experienced life so differently. Malnourished Jill was about half the size of Downstairs Jill.

The important step was that Malnourished Jill *allowed* her avatar to comfort her. No adults were able to do that. Malnourished Jill had no memory of an adult being helpful or even kind. Suddenly, not getting that downstairs avatar out of Lanner Street made sense. An adult, me, had been trying to show Malnourished Jill the future. Why the hell should Malnourished Jill believe any adult?

As that sisterly meeting went on, my guides cautioned patience with my avatar. I wanted to get Malnourished Jill out of that room immediately. I wanted to get her some food, a hot bath, and clothes that didn't make her look like she belonged in a coffin. But my guides cautioned me to let Malnourished Jill move when she was ready and let the medicine direct me.

Malnourished Jill didn't trust that Downstairs Jill avatar

could permanently improve things. She accepted the cuddling from that avatar but didn't want to enjoy it.

Joy taken away can be the emptiest feeling in the world.

Guide: We want to sit with Malnourished Jill. We just need to give her some time. Because this is entirely new to her, she has never been in this space before.

Jill: She doesn't know how to act.

Guide: Yeah.

Jill: Yeah, she doesn't know how to act. She doesn't trust it's going to stay good. She doesn't trust it's going to remain good. She can't get too used to things being good. It's not going to last. Even I feel bad for her.

Guide: Yeah, there you go.

Jill: I'm not going to like this. It is going to make it even harder when it gets taken away.

Guide: If I get attached here, I will have this ripped off of me later. So, this is a trust issue. Essentially there is no trust.

Jill: Why would there be trust? I mean, I know memories are selective and everything. I just can't remember good memories. I'm sure occasionally I smiled and had fun in my childhood. I just don't remember many of those times. So it makes sense. Like why would she trust? There is zero proof. Your pets get taken away. Your mom wants to commit suicide. Your mom wants to leave you with him. (Angry) Your mom wants to leave you behind with him. I don't think I ever forgave her for that.

183

———————

Through lots of rambling and conversation, I finally managed to get Malnourished Jill downstairs to eat at my little kiddie table in our 1970s dingy yellow and green kitchen.

Then my brain stopped.

When those two little girls looked where a door to the house used to be, they saw a wall.

There still wasn't a door they could use to leave the house.

At that point, I asked my guides for help. I was stuck in my childhood home.

Trapped.

I couldn't get out.

My guides knew this was the time for the mushrooms. The MDMA had done its job. I was very empathetic toward Malnourished Jill and wanted to help her. My mind needed a way to get her out of that house. Everything Malnourished Jill knew about that home had to be disrupted. My guides needed to find a way to teach Malnourished Jill, who lived deep in my subconscious, that Lanner Street wasn't her prison. Psilocybin (magic mushrooms) can distort perceptions and that is what Malnourished Jill needed. *She* needed to see her childhood home differently than she had ever seen it before.

Since we had talked about adding psilocybin to my therapy beforehand, my guide simply handed me a small bowl with some dried mushrooms. My guides told me to chew the mushrooms slowly while I thought about freeing Malnourished Jill from my childhood home. The mushrooms were going to do their best with a clear intention.

The next part of the journey, with the addition of mushrooms, started with the primary intention to get Malnourished Jill out of that awful house.

Chapter 44

Reparenting Psychedelic-Style

As the mushrooms kicked in, I needed to lie down. Of course, I was still chatting with my guides. My guides encouraged me to cover my eyes, relax into the medication, and let it do its job.

I resisted.

After all, they asked me to slow down and work on my scariest trapped emotions from when I was five.

This doesn't fill me with pride to admit, but part of my subconscious still fought the healing. All I had known my entire life was how I felt. How would I feel if life were different? Could I keep being successful and competent if I weren't constantly looking over my shoulder and hustling? Was my livelihood at stake if I healed and felt comfortable in my skin?

My guides knew I was being cagey by chatting and tried to guide my focus by asking me to "go into my body" to try and see where I felt the pain and trauma from when I was five. I couldn't specify a point in my body where the trauma was housed like some of the PTSD episodes I had experienced. This pain was much more in my head. It then filtered through my body.

I remember pointing to my head when I answered their questions about locating the childhood pain.

Thankfully, my guides were patient and persistent. I finally did as they asked and tried to quiet myself. Just like when I was a child, trying to soothe myself to sleep, I started to rub my feet together in endless figure eights. I pointed out to my guides that I seemed to be self-soothing.

Guide: I want to bring your attention there. See if you can bring your attention to your feet. Bring your attention to the rubbing. Allow yourself to experience this rubbing.

Jill: It calms me.

Guide: Yeah. See if you can invite yourself to go towards that. Go toward that calm. It seems to be something in the body that needs to be soothed. Just invite yourself to go toward that. Get curious about that. Curious about, "What is it in the body that needs to be soothed?" You are pointing to your head. Yeah. What is going on there?

Jill: I needed to be told that everything would be safe and ok. When I was little, I would rock in bed to get that anxiety out. But nobody ever came. That I remember.

Guide: What is the exact language? Everything is going to be ok? Is that what the body needs to hear?

Jill: Um… You're protected. You're safe. You're protected. You're not going to get hurt. This pain that is inside you. We will help you get rid of this pain inside you. You don't have to feel this way.

Guide: So, I want to see what happens if your therapist just offers that to you.

Therapist: Just to let you know—you are safe. Everything is going to be ok.

Jill: How do you know?

Therapist: I know.

Jill: No. No, you don't.

187

Therapist: It is hard to believe.

Guide: Who just showed up and said, "You don't know?"

Jill: Malnourished Jill.

Guide: Right. Great. What would she need to hear? What does she need to register that she has a healthy mom here?

Jill: She needs to go to another family. There is no other way around it. She needs to get out of that fucking house. And those fucking parents... She needs to be somewhere else, and she can't make that happen. (At this point in the treatment, the therapist I had worked with for years asked me if it was ok to hold my hand, and I agreed.)

Guide: I want you to really pay attention to this hand. Feel into it. What is happening to you? Can you feel this hand?

Jill: Support. Yeah, support. Thank you. This feels a little weird, but it is support. This is what never came. I feel like a big, giant dork right now.

Therapist: Beautiful.

Guide: Those are her inner protectors again. Let's let poor Malnourished Jill that never got this, have this.

Jill: Boy, I am so uncomfortable with this.

Guide: So just check in with that. Check in with that. Where is that discomfort? Where in the body is it?

Jill: I feel like I am being too inconvenient. I feel like I am being too much. I'm too much trouble.

Therapist: Yeah. That is kind of the story she made up right? She must be too much trouble.

Jill: She must be too much trouble. Cause they

188

never did this.

Therapist: Right. Or she would have gotten what she needed. She must have been too much.

Guide: So now we can reframe it. She wasn't too much. They just didn't know how to love.

Jill: Yeah.

———

My guides used MDMA, psilocybin, and reparenting strategies to reframe my child-centric beliefs that I wasn't *enough* to be loved. Did it feel awkward? Oh yeah. Even with my enhanced state with two psychedelics in my system, I was extremely uncomfortable with the kindness my therapist gave me. I didn't trust that another adult wouldn't have an ulterior motive when interacting with me.

My discomfort made sense because for me to get calm reassurance from anyone resembling a parental figure was a new experience. This work was necessary to break down the *adults can't be trusted* walls that my inner five-year-old had crafted.

I'm not saying I understood that at the time. At the time, I didn't trust it. Thank goodness for the psychedelics and months of work that allowed me to relax enough and trust my guides to accept this bit of re-parenting.

Chapter 45

I'm Done

As the parental reframing was happening, my mind continued to fight.

My parents jerked me around too many times, so I didn't believe that anything remotely parental could be trusted.

————

Jill: If I trust you, how do I know you will not go away?

Therapist: How would I go away? What would that look like?

Jill: I don't know. Stop this treatment? Be disappointed it didn't work?

Therapist: So, I could just abandon ship? Or I would say, "You screwed up. I don't want to do this anymore since you disappointed me."

Jill: Yeah. What need do you have? Why are you doing this? What am I not going to be able to fulfill for you?

Therapist: Right. It's like some sort of setup. This is actually for me, and you will screw it up. Then you aren't going to get what you need.

Jill: Yeah.

Therapist: Everything good is going to get taken away.

Jill: Yes. When I least expect it. And I wanted to be over that fear at the end of the second journey. But I'm not. But if everything gets lost a third time, I will just give up. I don't have any more energy to fight it. If the universe wants to crap on me, the universe will be able to do it this time around. *I'm done.*

This "I'm done" was the primary reason I worked so hard for over a year in this treatment. When I agreed to MDMA initially, I was borderline suicidal. I never fully admitted it in any of our sessions, but I know my therapist had a hunch. A patient sitting on her couch can only say "I'm done" so many times until the meaning is clear.

I had been living my life racing to safety with a heavy rucksack on my back, constantly looking over my shoulder, and I couldn't get to the finish line. I was bone tired. No amount of planning or work had gotten me feeling even remotely secure. I could not take another devastating *starting over from scratch* disaster. I started too many times to count throughout my childhood. Then I did it at sixteen, I did it at nineteen, and I did it at forty-six when Carl died. I still questioned if I had the potential for a happy future in front of me.

I looked happy and confident, but inside, I was exhausted. I had no interest in living through another upheaval. All I had left was my financial security and my health. If one of those went sideways, I would take the universe's hint and bow out. *I was done.*

Guide: I am going to call that surrender. That's good.
Jill: That's good?

Guide: Surrender in that you can let life in. You no longer resist the stream of life and where it will take you. You can even let go of the narrative that it will be terrible or horrible or ugly.

Jill: Or life being so much work. Life is just going to be more and more work. Can there be life without doing a ton of work?

Guide: You can surrender to life, and life will guide you. You see, the thing is in every moment we are going into the mystery of life. I still haven't met anyone with a crystal ball who can tell me exactly what will happen next. The moment I became clear that there was mystery to life, and it was inevitable, then I had a choice. I could be scared of the mystery and be in a place of fear, or I could get curious. I could be like a child waking up every day in the summer when there is no school. I don't know how the day will go, but I'll find out! Life is still a mystery, but it is so much lighter when I am not scared of it. It is so much more amazing just to discover the things that show up in life.

Jill: Yeah, I guess I was always scared of not knowing what would come next.

Therapist: How could you not be?

Chapter 46

Busting Open Lanner Street

At this point, we were almost four hours into the journey, and the psilocybin was kicking in. I vaguely remember commenting on beautiful flashes of light and wonderful shapes because I was very relaxed. It was like I could watch my mind staging a Salvador Dalí-like show. Many colorful images morphed and moved at their own pace behind my closed eyelids.

My guides and I agreed it was time to try to get the Jills out of the Lanner Street house. They again encouraged me to get quiet to let the medicine work. Fortunately for my guides, but not fortunate for explaining this part of the healing, I finally listened and put on my eye mask and settled myself under the covers. I didn't talk about how my childhood house simply fell apart while it happened, but the memory was so vivid that I had no trouble telling my guides about it when I came out of that part of the journey.

•••••••

I remember Malnourished Jill and Healthy Jill were sitting at my kiddie table in the 1970s kitchen. Then all the colors, furniture, and walls fell away. It was like when I didn't use enough icing on a gingerbread house I tried to make years ago. A complete side of the house fell over because I didn't seal the edges well enough. That was how the walls of my childhood home all fell away. They seemed to move outward and downward—essentially turning upside down.

As the house walls fell, I suddenly watched everything through Malnourished Jill's eyes. I became that starving, beaten-up little girl. The Healthy Jill avatar had disappeared.

Then I was surrounded by simple black space. I was aware the house was still there, but it was changing—being stripped away of what made it that particular house. I wasn't scared at all while I watched this happen. In fact, I looked around, interested in what was happening, and was surprised at how lovely the color black was.

Then, while I stood in the kitchen that no longer had walls, the floor started to come apart. I stood on a kitchen tile while the floor separated, and turned black, while each tile looked like an individual platform. The kitchen seemed to turn itself inside out, and I was still on a tile, and I felt I could jump to the other tile platforms if I wanted. It was like a giant, black blooming onion where each onion spear had a standing platform.

As I stood there, I saw the shiny black house, with all those little empty tile platforms, just fall away. The house just opened and turned itself inside out so I could get out. The house no longer was my inner child's prison.

Then I was in a lovely garden in the blink of

an eye. The house was gone, and I sat in a quiet, private backyard that was lush with tall trees, colorful flowers, and green grass. That garden, most importantly, had no adults. My parents weren't part of this experience at all. I, as Malnourished Jill, was in a healthy garden with birds chirping and the sun warming my face. With its internal darkness and dread, that house was gone, and I was outside, breathing fresh air with no sense of danger.

●●●●●●●●

My guides joked a bit about what that garden was like. They threw some imagery in it for me, but I pretty much stuck to a lovely lounge chair and a cool glass of water. I remember, even then, being full of gratitude that I was safe. I wasn't going to push it by asking for even a toothpick Kool-Aid cherry popsicle that had been a summer treat on warm afternoons.

I would never have guessed where my internal sense of isolation and not belonging came from. I always blamed it on not having a family. After this experience, it was clear that the isolation I felt as an adult stemmed from that little five-year-old Malnourished Jill who was trapped in her childhood bedroom. I carried her inside my head my entire adult life. After rescuing her during this journey, the shedding of her fear gave me an almost immediate bounce in my step.

I wasn't alone in this world.

I didn't have to stay huddled in that drab room surrounded by angry patriarchal cruelty. There wasn't something big and dangerous lurking beyond the door to my childhood room. That room didn't exist anymore.

When people claim that psychedelic-assisted psychotherapy is some crazy number of talk therapy years boiled down to a crazy small number of journey hours, they reference this kind of experience. I'm not sure I would ever have been able to achieve this level of healing without directly accessing my subconscious. And let me be clear, I would never have accessed this deep fear-filled trauma space in my mind if not for the months of work, the prior journeys, the trust I had in my guides, and MDMA in my system making me feel safe.

The months and months of talk therapy work, my skilled guides, the medication, and my dedication to doing the hard, uncomfortable work were all partners in this breakthrough.

Chapter 47

Just Jill

Interestingly, the medicine didn't have me stay in that garden long because it was ready to do more work!

There was a long pause while I processed being in that lovely garden. Then, entirely by surprise, I shared a memory from a trip to Costa Rica with my guides.

●●●●●●●

I was lucky enough to travel as a chaperone for my school district's foreign language trips before I had the resources to travel on vacations. One of the trips was to beautiful Costa Rica. As one can imagine, there was minimal downtime while chaperoning a bunch of teenagers.

But one afternoon, we had time to address our jet lag, and we were on this isolated, beautiful seaside property, so there weren't too many ways kids could get into trouble. It was one of the safest places I have ever been.

That afternoon, I took a book, found a shady hammock, flipped off my sandals, and welcomed the ocean breeze. I relaxed completely. I had zero responsibilities for an hour or so.

The weather was lovely, and wild monkeys

were full of shenanigans in the trees above. It was one of the few times in my life where I could just be me, enjoy what I was doing and where I was.

There was no avatar. There was no "responsible Jill" doing her leadership thing. I didn't have to be anything for someone else.

I was just Jill getting to relax and not co-dependently taking care of anyone else.

●●●●●●●●

———————

Jill: I could just *be* when I was in the hammock.
Therapist: Could you just be what?
Guide: You could be without all the parts of you "doing?"
Jill: There is always a list. Carl used to say, "Stop making things up. Things are ok. You don't have to be this busy." And I was like, no, can't you see everything that needs to be done? It is hard to settle.
Guide: Somewhere in you, there is balance. Somewhere in there is, "There is stuff to do. Can't you see?" But there is also a freedom that you don't have to always be in action out of compulsion. I think that is what Carl is talking about. You feel like you always have to be doing something. What is that about?
Jill: It is the only thing I have. When I get quiet, I don't have anything else.
Guide: Yeah. So, let's just see, if for a moment, if you can sit there with nothing and see what happens

next.

Jill: Nothing happened.

Guide: Yeah, so then can you take that in? Take in this quiet moment where nothing happened? There was no concern or worry. You are just here. What are you thinking that makes you nod?

Jill: Someone is taking away the cement around me. Chopping off the dried, old cement that was holding me. And I was saying, "Yes, do it. I can't do it. I need help."

———————

The mushrooms showed me I needed to think differently from a common image I used at work all the time. I often described my experience of doing long and arduous work tasks as having to "walk through dried cement." When I read the transcript, I smiled because the medicine broke away the dried cement of my thinking. It was clear that once my inner five-year-old was out of my childhood home, I didn't always have to be struggling to survive. I didn't have to be in motion to be safe. My *stay on the ball* thinking had been so ingrained and such a part of my life. I needed help to relax. As clearly as the medicine opened my home to free me, it also chiseled away at my deeply held survival tactic of running on all cylinders 24/7.

Chapter 48

Defining Myself

The transcript showed, for the rest of the afternoon, while coming down from the medication, I talked about the same themes of letting go of Carl, letting someone else into my heart, and not being afraid of the next chapter in my life. I think it is telling that there was no more mention of that little Malnourished Jill as she had been freed! I rehashed a few oldies but goodies about not feeling good enough and not loving my parents. I think it was just the medicine's way of coating those feelings to work on them during my integration.

We did all the usual post journey return to the real-world things. We had some snacks, drank water, and took a grounding walk outside. My guides were thrilled with the day and felt confident we had freed me from my childhood home. I didn't remember much, and I was still fascinated that I was with them for about eight hours, while it felt like thirty minutes.

The next day, I had a big hangover, so I took care of myself and tried to sleep as much as possible. I also listened to the transcript when I was awake because I was so curious. But it was eight hours long, so there was a lot to get through!

I was also a little scared. You see, my internal voice that I had heard consistently after the first and second journey was silent.

I panicked and thought maybe the dosage of the MDMA was off or something? Perhaps my brain wasn't responding anymore? What if the mushrooms shut down my inner voice? What if all the preparation work was for nothing?

Luckily, the next day, things started to fall into place again. Not only did my inner voice come back, but I had some great visualizations with my healing. The integration process after having psilocybin was different from the other two MDMA journeys. I feel like this last journey is the classic thing people expect when I talk about psychedelic-assisted psychotherapy. Finally, I had some funky stories to tell!

First, I heard the voice come back strong after listening to a portion of the transcript where I talked about never feeling good enough to be loved. My inner voice was having none of it!

> **Inner Voice:** You don't listen to any of his (my father's) bullshit, right? Why the heck are you listening to that shit? There is no reason to carry his definition of you anymore. *You* get to define who you are.

And as I walked Sadie, I started to see myself as a caring, loving, and strong person who is *not* alone and *will not* be alone moving forward.

Shedding the idea that I was alone was monumental. But there wasn't anyone clapping. There was no big shindig. No announcer gave me an award. I walked back to the house with Sadie like I had done so many times before but with a much lighter step.

Instead, there was a lovely feeling of getting rid of uncomfortable layers. I had the welcoming feeling of coming into a warm home and shrugging off a snow-covered coat. I was able to shake off thoughts and emotions that didn't serve me.

The shift might have been quiet, but it was mighty.

Chapter 49

Visualization Healing

Later that night, when I got quiet, I continued my integration work with some amazing visualizations about getting out of the Lanner Street house. There was a marked difference between the integration work from MDMA-only journeys and one with a touch of psilocybin added. My MDMA journeys and integration work had primarily concentrated on voice and memories.

This psilocybin-added journey, and the subsequent integration, had much more visualization work as part of the healing process. Since it was so different from the last two integrations, I was slightly concerned because I didn't know if I was hallucinating. But I checked in with my guides and described what I saw. The images were very much like daydreams. There was no question that what I was seeing was firmly in my mind, and I had no difficulty determining what was real versus my mind's activity. My guides had no concerns and told me to enjoy the process. I followed their advice, and I felt my creativity and imagination waking up. I know those aspects of my personality had been dampened big time with Carl's passing.

This process didn't wait for Sadie's walks. For instance, the first significant visualization started when I was sitting on the couch journaling. In my mind, I saw four Jills at different ages in the Lanner Street house. We were all in the pretty downstairs bedroom I had mentally created months before. I pictured Adult Jill, the avatar Downstairs

Jill, a seven-year-old Jill, and Malnourished Jill. I
remember being surprised that the house was still standing
as I remembered it disintegrating during the journey.

Then the most amazing thing happened. My seven-year-
old Jill held Malnourished Jill's hand, and they walked out
of that house together. Suddenly the door that had been
there in real life appeared, and they walked through it. I
remember smiling when they got to the house's driveway!

Adult Jill and Downstairs Jill simply watched from the
house door. We were ready to help if needed, but I
instinctively knew that Malnourished Jill didn't trust adults
yet. It seemed natural that seven-year-old Jill, who had
gotten out of that room years before, appeared to help her. I
was eight years old when I started to live with my father
and his girlfriend, so I think my mind purposely chose an
age where I had felt safe with relatives.

I remember feeling so calm and free watching this
visualization. The heaviness of being trapped in that house
wasn't there anymore. In my gratitude, I looked out past the
driveway to see marshmallow, fluffy, person-shaped
energies surrounding us. It was like there wasn't a
neighborhood beyond my childhood driveway. Instead,
there was this cocoon of loving spiritual energy that
protected those two little girls. The figures were billowy
and soft, sending oodles of love and kindness. They
collectively sent the message, "You are not alone."

And guess who was right in front? The only figure, in a
form I could recognize, was Carl grinning from ear to ear.
Everyone who knew him will smile to hear he was in his
classic uniform of jeans and a T-shirt.

Malnourished Jill couldn't believe it, and she let those
energies crowd around her in their billowy softness. One
even picked her up and held her closer to the sun. That

embrace was the start of her nourishment.

Then the two little girls started to spin and play in the bright, warm sunshine. Sidewalk chalk and roller skates appeared, and they created little chalk-drawn paths for their skating city. There was food and clothing on both sides of the driveway.

It was freedom. The two little girls were thrilled with basic food, clothing, and the security of knowing neither parent was around.

Then I found it fascinating that a little tent showed up in the driveway. I guessed because that seven-year-old Jill and Malnourished Jill didn't know where to go? That seven-year-old had been shuffled to various relatives, so it made sense she didn't have a real idea of where to head. Suddenly a tent with some comfortable beds magically appeared. In my journal, I wondered if Malnourished Jill just needed a little time to acclimate to being out of that house. For her it was probably like seeing a sunny day peak through blackout curtains. She needed a little time to adjust to the world outside of the room where she had been trapped for so long.

I was right. That little girl just needed a little time and grew rapidly in the coming days!

Chapter 50

Give Jill Time

The next day during Sadie's walk, with the warm sun shining, I continued to free my inner five-year-old by giving my imagination the space to do what it wanted.

I easily pictured seven-year-old and Malnourished Jill in the driveway. They were happy, laughing, and playing silly sidewalk chalk games. Suddenly, Malnourished Jill stood still, looked around, and magically flew above the Lanner Street house. As she soared into the air, she realized the house no longer had a second level. Her little prison just didn't exist.

I smiled as I walked behind Sadie because I felt an amazing sense of freedom. Little Malnourished Jill says no to society's pull that family is everything. She gets to say, "Nope, nadda, I'm outta here!" She doesn't have to stay anywhere near that house anymore. She gets to leave her parents' hope-destroying life behind.

I know this might sound sad to anyone with a fantastic family, but for me, who hadn't experienced love and kindness from family members, not feeling tied to my abusive father and depressed mother was wonderful.

Malnourished Jill landed back on the driveway and hugged seven-year-old Jill. Then, they held hands and simply walked away from the house. When they got to the sidewalk, they stopped, looked around and turned right.

In real life, that turn leads to a road that quickly turns into eight-lane Route 1. But instead of noisy cars whizzing by on a busy highway, the girls found themselves on a hill overlooking the ocean. I remember the blue waters with light dancing on the waves. I felt their sense of wonder looking at the expanse of water that met the horizon.

Then I joined them and stood to the side. They allowed me to stand with them. They allowed an adult to be with them.

It was surreal to see myself at seven and a much shorter Malnourished Jill looking at the horizon. I turned to the water to see what captured their attention. The shining blue water and gentle waves beckoned with the promise of happier days ahead.

Chapter 51

Time to Grow

Suddenly, I felt Malnourished Jill tugging on my hand and asking to be picked up. She wanted to see the ocean from my perspective. I picked her up, noticed how light she was for a five-year-old and gently asked her:

> **Jill**: Why do you still look so sickly?
> **Malnourished Jill:** I just need a little time. I'm a kid. I need to grow.

And with that, I understood to let her grow at her own pace, not rush things, and make sure that she got lots of love and hugs. I was on the road to re-parent myself.

I was conscientious about paying attention to my body's signals in the coming days. I realized that whenever my brain got super fuzzy, it was Malnourished Jill's way of tugging on my hand. She took baby steps learning about the world.

I listened and always slowed down when I felt her presence. And for maybe the first time in my life, by paying attention to the needs of my inner five-year-old, I put myself first.

Chapter 52

Simply Jill

This last journey happened to be scheduled five days before my birthday. Fellow adults who had crappy childhood birthday experiences know that those days, regardless of how much fun they might be as an adult, carry sadness-tinged memories. My birthday, my entire life, was always a bit of a trigger for empty and sad emotions to swirl in my head.

In my journal the day before my birthday, I wrote about looking forward to my birthday! I was happy that I had made it this far. Lots of boot camp classes allowed me to keep moving around well for my age with just a few pesky creaks from my knees. But what was subtle and massive at the same time was that the empty feeling I always had in the pit of my stomach was gone. I had an exciting sense of wholeness. It wasn't as simple as feeling full after a big meal, but that was the best way to describe it to my friends who didn't understand the isolation I had felt deep inside me my entire life.

There was no ear-splitting drum roll.

There was no queued audience applause.

There was no gold-plated sparkling trophy.

I just noticed that I didn't feel empty anymore. I felt full of *me*. I was simply Jill.

I was an individual who could take up space in this world without always thinking she didn't belong because she didn't have parents who loved her. Malnourished Jill taught me why I had those terrible thinking patterns! If she didn't have that essential thing—love from her parents—what did she have? Well, on this day, the day before my birthday, you know what she and I had? We had me as an adult who could finally love herself.

It was both subtle and monumental at the same time.

There was a fundamental shift in how I thought about myself. It was almost like every cell of my body had been relieved of my childhood baggage. The fear and shame of my childhood were no longer in my bones. And who was I? Well, I was a loving and competent person who broke my family's trauma cycle. I was dedicated to working on my healing to make the next chapter of my life happy.

Ironically, some parts of this book were difficult to write because I now feel whole. This book wouldn't have been possible without my journals because I am not the person I was at the start of this therapy. I don't live constantly looking over my shoulder. I'm comfortable with taking up space in the world now. I know the universe has been kind to me.

When I told my therapist how difficult it was to remember the feelings of isolation and worthlessness that had plagued me my entire life, she wasn't surprised. She said, "Of course! Do you think a butterfly spends time remembering what it was like as a caterpillar?"

Chapter 53

Learning Security

The following day, or the day before my birthday, I was stuck spring cleaning. But I felt wonderfully comfortable doing the routine house chores and enjoyed getting some of the winter clutter organized. I wasn't concerned about spending the weekday of my birthday alone. I had planned this week for my brain to relax and respond to the treatment. It was a complete shock not to feel alone and sad during my birthday week while I puttered around the house.

That newly freed Malnourished Jill looked adorable in modern kid clothes with a bit of glitter on her shirt. She had gained weight and grown a few inches. Her hair was shiny brown in a high ponytail that brushed her shoulders. She was suddenly confident and showed up next to me while I ran errands. I had this feeling that my younger self was enjoying seeing my adult life. There wasn't any formal goodbye to Lanner Street. She just started hanging out with me as she learned about life from an adult who had her shit together and didn't tolerate drama. I delighted in seeing her growing healthier and happier by the day.

One specific event stood out in my journals. I felt her presence once when I went food shopping. I felt her eyes on me as I took items off the shelves. I wondered about that, and when I got to the checkout line, she appeared next to me with eyes wide and an overly concerned look on her face. She watched me intently with a worried frown on her face as I paid for groceries. I found it curious, and as I walked out of the store, I remembered one of the times my mother tried to escape my father.

●●●●●●●●

I think I might have been four. My mother had hurriedly packed us a bag and shuttled me into the car. We went to the local Kmart or something, and I remember we collected a cart full of items. I was excited because there was a pair of shoes I wanted in the cart.

When we got to the checkout line, my mother's credit card got declined. Either my father figured out she was trying to leave him, and he put a hold on the card, or the card was maxed out. That card was my mother's lifeline to try and start fresh.

I remember being disappointed that I couldn't get a pair of shoes. I didn't understand what was happening at the time. But I'll never forget my mother's tears as we walked through the check-out line, and she left the entire cart behind. I remember understanding that whatever was going on was much bigger than my shoes, so I stayed quiet.

I can only imagine how my mother felt, knowing that the moment the clerk declined the purchases, she had to go back to that monster.

●●●●●●●

It made sense why that little girl so keenly watched me pay the grocery bill. That memory explained why she visibly relaxed as we walked out of the store. She knew she didn't have to go back to Lanner Street and my father. I knew she was fine when she wandered away as I packed the car. She acted like every kid getting out of doing tedious chores instead of double and triple-checking that the groceries were in the car.

I didn't write about her for the rest of the day. I think she was happy to check off *there is money to buy stuff, I'm safe* from her internal checklist.

Chapter 54

The End, For Now

The next few days I spent transcribing the journey. My focus was on listening to how my mind worked while the medication did its thing.

A few days after my birthday, I mentioned in my journal that while I was walking Sadie, Malnourished Jill, who had gotten healthy, was suddenly curled up in my belly. I thought and still think, that was a little weird. I had this feeling that she just always wanted to be with me. She trusted me. She knew we would have a good life.

But honestly, I thought this was taking integration just a little too far.

I checked in with my guides, and they didn't see an issue. They encouraged me to stay mindful and aware of the process. About three weeks later, Malnourished Jill thoroughly blended into me. I didn't imagine her as a separate person or curled up in my belly any longer.

I also noticed that my hair twirling and lip biting were down significantly. They weren't gone, which was a bit of a disappointment, but I was more aware of those behaviors, which allowed me to curb them more than ever before. I guess that as much as they were trauma responses, they became part of my self-soothing muscle memory since I have been doing them for so long. I decided to follow the same advice with those behaviors as my therapist suggested with how to treat Malnourished Jill's bonding with me. I was to stay mindful and aware of my behaviors to understand them more.

I've struggled a bit with where to end my story because I am a work in progress. Every day I make steps forward. I still reshape how I think about my fears and long-held thoughts. Every day I get stronger and more familiar with my strong and loving self. It is lovely getting to know myself now.

I no longer qualify for a PTSD diagnosis. I've ended the cycle of family trauma that I inherited from my parents.

The point of sharing my healing story was to show there is help for childhood trauma-induced PTSD sufferers. I think I've done that. I've allowed you, the reader, into my brain, with all of its weirdness, to validate how untreated trauma manifests into our adult behavior. Most importantly, healing can happen with trusted guides, patients putting the time into unraveling the origins of deep emotional pain, and professionally administered psychedelics.

As I looked back at the year's journeys, it seemed like I added warmth to my life. In the beginning, when that horrendous panic attack took me to my therapist's couch, my life was like a picture that was so glaring with fear that I could only see the outlines of how to live. I was just living a skeletal life of dread from my early childhood trauma. I wasn't really living.

As the year of my healing progressed, I started to see my life from a different perspective, and the picture I had of myself, and the future, became tinted. It started slowly with muted tones for sure, but at the end of the year, the colors amplified, and I felt a new richness inside of me that replaced most of that blinding fear.

I no longer felt that the universe was out to get me. I knew I had a future ahead of me.

Healing from trauma is not like flipping off a light

switch, though. While I was thrilled I no longer qualified for a PTSD diagnosis, months later I asked my guides for one more journey.

I had a nightmare that brought forth a deep fear of men, and I couldn't talk therapy my way out of it.

That is another story for another day. I mention it because this kind of healing requires persistence and deep dives into pain. I didn't know I had more levels of trauma until my subconscious knocked on my door months after the third journey. Every day I keep learning more about myself.

I started this book by talking about Carl's death. With his loss, all my childhood shit swirled into a cacophony of fear and dread about the future. Then eighteen months after his passing, I hit my tolerance limit with that work email that sent me over the edge into that dizzying panic attack. With the help of psychedelic-assisted psychotherapy and two amazing guides, I healed enough to share my story of overcoming childhood trauma-induced PTSD. I wrote the book to offer hope to others who inherited trauma passed down from prior generations. I feel so tremendously lucky to have healed and I hope continued research will bring more people relief in the future.

I now know the universe works in strange and winding ways. While his death closed the door on our relationship, it led me to an opportunity to release decades-old trauma.

My year-long journey of healing was a tremendous fucking door to open!

References

Bessel van der Kolk, M.D. The Body Keeps the Score: Brain, Mind, and Body in the Healing of Trauma. New York: Penguin Books, 2015.

About the Author
JillSitnick.com

In her 26-year career in educational technology, Jill Sitnick has been an educator, Supervisor of Instructional Technology, and a Microsoft Program Manager and Education Executive.

At her core, she is a teacher known for her ability to simplify complex issues using storytelling to connect people to innovative ideas.

Most recently she is the author of *Rescuing Jill, How MDMA, with a Dash of Magic Mushrooms, Healed my Childhood Trauma-Induced PTSD*. Jill shared her experience with PTSD to explain her healing with psychedelic-assisted psychotherapy. She is a strong advocate for more research into psychedelics for mental health issues in the hopes of giving more people the opportunity to heal.

Jill lives in Pennsylvania with her clingy dog, who keeps the house safe from a litany of sketchy squirrels.

www.ingramcontent.com/pod-product-compliance
Lightning Source LLC
Chambersburg PA
CBHW062130020426
42335CB00013B/1161